Superfoods

The Best Foods
for Top Nutrition

2023 Report

A Special Report published by
the editors of *Environmental Nutrition*

Superfoods: The Best Foods for Top Nutrition

Author: Sharon Palmer MSFS, RDN
Update Author: Kristen N. Smith, PhD, RDN, LD
Creative Director, Belvoir Media Group: Judi Crouse
Belvoir Editor: Dawn Bialy
Production: Mary Francis McGavic

Publisher, Belvoir Media Group: Timothy H. Cole
Executive Editor, Book Division, Belvoir Media Group: Lynn Russo

Print ISBN 978-1-941937-00-6
Digital ISBN 978-1-941937-99-0

To order additional copies of this report or for customer-service questions, please call 877-300-0253, or write: Health Special Reports, 535 Connecticut Avenue, Norwalk, CT 06854-1713.

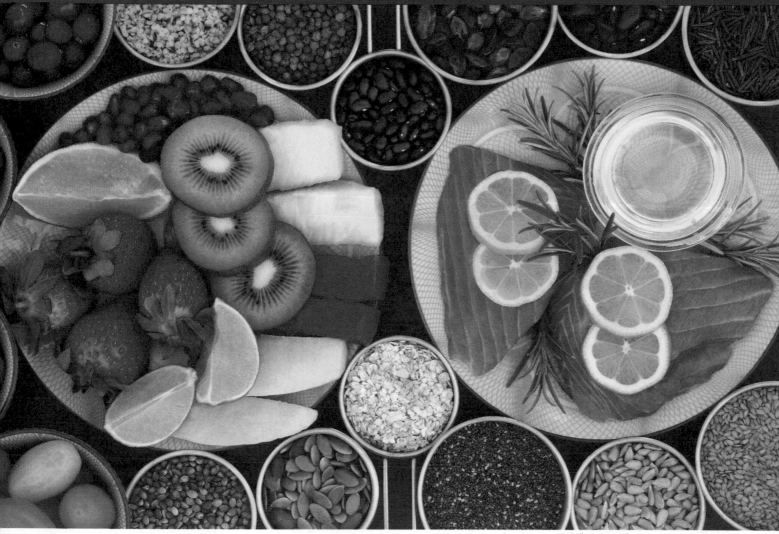

© Marilyna | Dreamstime

This Special Report on superfoods is brought to you by the editors of *Environmental Nutrition*, an authoritative, trusted nutrition newsletter for both consumers and health-care professionals.

The connection between your health and your diet is indisputable. Poor-quality diets that lack important nutrients contribute to many of the leading causes of death in the United States, including heart disease, stroke and cerebrovascular disease, many types of cancer, and diabetes.

On one hand, we're fortunate to have easy access to an enormous amount of information via our computers and smartphones. On the other hand, with so much information at our fingertips, it can be difficult to determine which sources are reputable and which are not.

This Special Report cuts through the confusion and tells you about the nutrition you need for optimum health. The information in these pages is based on research conducted by nutrition experts and published in the most respected medical and nutrition journals. You'll learn which proteins, grains, vegetables, fruits, and other foods are highest in the nutrients that provide proven health benefits. You'll also get smart shopping strategies and tips that make it a breeze to eat healthfully at home. And we give you delicious recipes that will make it easy to get superfoods onto your plate.

Healthy eating doesn't have to be complicated. In fact, it's simple: If you follow the guidance provided in this Special Report, you will improve your diet and your health every day.

TABLE OF CONTENTS

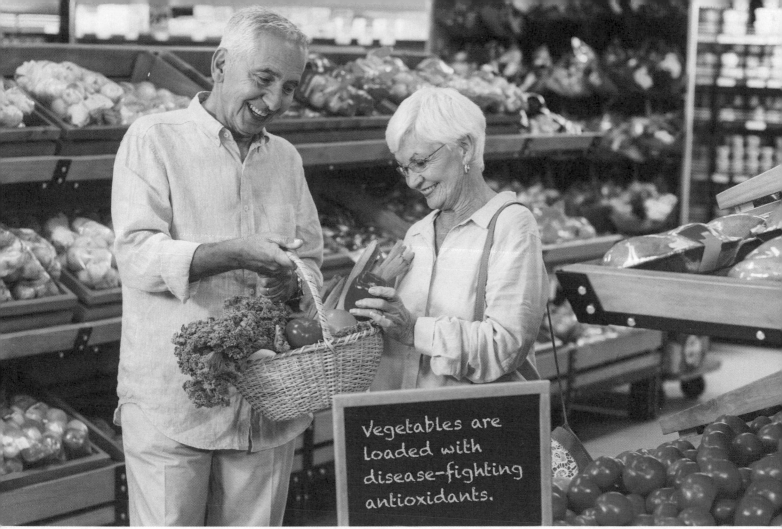

© Wavebreakmediamicro | Dreamstime

New Findings

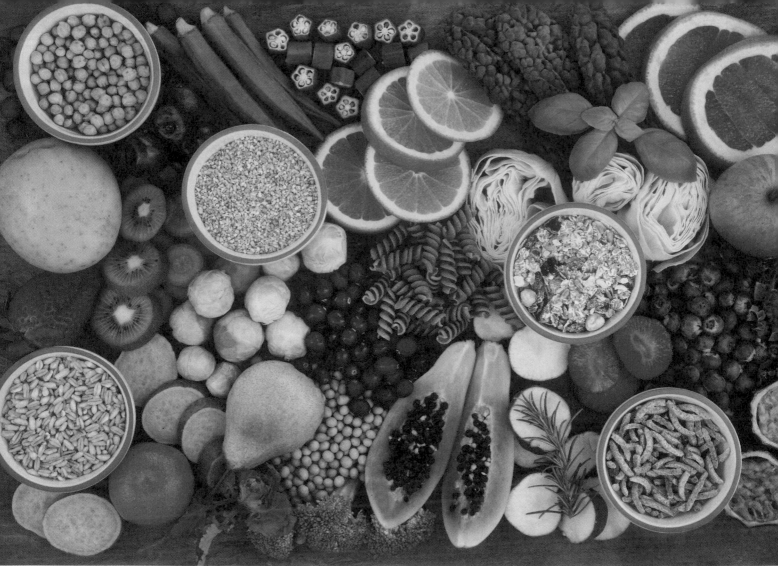

A diet that supports good health focuses on foods that are packed with a variety of nutrients.

1 Superfoods

Making conscious, careful choices about what you put on your plate is one of the most important things you can do to preserve and protect your health. As researchers continue to investigate some of the most prevalent diseases facing society today, it's becoming clearer that there's a direct link between what you eat and how you feel. In fact, risks for the majority of chronic diseases (including cardiovascular disease, various types of cancer, type 2 diabetes, osteoporosis, and Alzheimer's disease) decrease significantly when you choose a lifestyle that includes following a healthy, balanced diet, incorporating regular exercise into your routine, getting an adequate amount of restful sleep, consuming moderate amounts of alcohol (or none), and avoiding tobacco use.

If you're like most people, your interest in taking better care of your health has grown as you've gotten older. This isn't surprising, since advancing age is the most common risk factor for the vast majority of chronic diseases. Fortunately, our knowledge about the relationship between diet and health has also grown, so it's now easier than ever to get science-based information and guidance about what to eat for better health.

The environment is another factor that has a growing influence on the dietary choices we make. As the damaging impacts of climate change become clearer, greater emphasis has been put on selecting foods with the smallest carbon footprint (meaning that the least amount of carbon dioxide is emitted during the production of those foods). When you make dietary choices that protect the environment—plant-based, whole or minimally processed foods—you're simultaneously choosing the same types of foods that offer the most protection for your health.

As the amount of information about our diet's impact on our bodies and our planet has grown, so, too, has the number of theories about which dietary patterns are best. For example, you may read that you will be healthier if you stop eating bread, pasta, and grains, but your sister tells you she's heard that cutting back on fat is the healthiest dietary strategy. How do you know which to believe—or if either one is accurate or even safe? That's where this report comes in: It provides you with information that is based on hundreds of high-quality scientific studies and consensus reports, rather than on one person's or group's opinion. As you read this report, you can be confident that you are getting the knowledge you need to choose the foods that have been shown to promote optimal health and longevity.

The Disease Process

Scientists now understand that two common conditions, chronic inflammation and oxidative stress, are at the root of many chronic diseases, especially those associated with aging. Learning about what causes these conditions will help you gain an understanding of how to alter your diet for better health.

Acute, short-term inflammation is a sign that your body's natural defense system is working. Acute inflammation is activated any time your body experiences injury or trauma, such as a cut, an infection, or a broken bone. The injury sends an automatic signal that sets off defense mechanisms designed to protect you. This defense includes increased blood flow that brings macrophages (cells that ingest dead or damaged cells, bacteria, and other substances that may cause harm) to the area of injury. When this occurs, your skin may become hot, red, and/or swollen. Once the threat has been fought off successfully, the inflammatory response shuts off.

However, sometimes, the body's inflammatory reaction fails to shut off, or it becomes activated when there is no external, identifiable trigger. When the inflammatory response remains turned on for weeks, months, or even years, it is referred to as chronic inflammation; this type of inflammation can have damaging rather than protective effects. Virtually every organ and system in your body—your heart, brain, nervous system, lungs, kidneys, liver, pancreas, skin, joints, and digestive system—can be harmed by chronic inflammation.

Oxidative stress occurs when the number of unstable molecules called free radicals in your body exceeds your body's ability to neutralize them. Free radicals are a byproduct of your body's metabolic processes, but they also form in response to environmental contaminants, such as tobacco smoke, pollution, pesticides, heavy metals, radiation, and other toxins. Over time, oxidative stress can lead to diseases of aging. Oxidative stress and inflammation go hand in hand—oxidative stress causes inflammation, and inflammation causes oxidative stress.

Food as Medicine

Think of your kitchen as nature's medicine cabinet. The foods you choose to nourish your body can help protect you from the diseases of aging. For centuries, cultures around the world have used certain foods to treat illness and disease. Some substances in foods can help counter chronic inflammation and oxidative stress; in effect, they can act as medicine that helps protect your health.

A diet that is comprised of whole plant foods, healthful carbohydrates and fats, and moderate amounts of lean protein has anti-inflammatory effects. This dietary pattern is rich in antioxidant compounds, which help neutralize free radicals and reduce oxidative stress. This type of eating pattern is what most health organizations, including the American Heart Association, the Academy of Nutrition and Dietetics, and the American Institute for Cancer Research, recommend for optimal health.

Conversely, poor food choices can promote illness and disease. Studies have shown that diets high in refined grains (such as white flour), processed meats, added sugars, and saturated fats and low in whole grains, pulses, fruits, vegetables, healthy fats, and fish appear to activate the body's inflammatory response. Often, this dietary pattern is referred to as the "Western diet" or "SAD" (Standard American Diet)—an eating pattern typically found in industrialized nations, such as the United States, that contains more highly processed and fast foods and fewer whole plant foods. This eating pattern is generally high in calories, saturated fat, sodium, and added sugars, and lower in vitamins, minerals, healthy fats, fiber, and phytochemicals.

The Western diet has been associated with the development of many conditions, including hypertension, high LDL ("bad") cholesterol, elevated blood glucose, obesity, and a weakened immune system, that can cause or contribute to many types of chronic diseases, including diabetes, heart and vascular diseases, rheumatoid arthritis, cancer, and even impaired brain function. This eating pattern also has a high carbon footprint (meaning that the production of these foods creates a large amount of greenhouse gases, primarily carbon dioxide, that are released into the atmosphere) compared to more healthful eating patterns.

The Healthiest Eating Patterns

The 2020–2025 *Dietary Guidelines for Americans*, an authoritative guide on healthy eating jointly produced by the U.S. Department of Agriculture and the U.S. Department of Health & Human Services, is updated every five years to reflect the most recent scientific findings about the impact of diet and nutrition on health. Based on these findings, a panel of the nation's top nutrition experts prepares a report, which is then interpreted into the official set of dietary guidelines.

In the 2020–2025 *Dietary Guidelines for Americans*, dietary recommendations are included for all life stages, from infants to seniors, stressing that it's never too early or too late to follow a healthy dietary pattern. It also calls for customizing nutrient-dense foods and beverages to reflect preferences, cultural traditions, and budgetary considerations. Culturally relevant foods are included in all food groups, so you can create a nutrient-dense diet that meets your own food preferences based on your heritage. Many Asian dishes, for example, contain a variety of vegetables, along with whole grains and plant-based proteins.

The guidelines, which emphasize that every bite counts, recommend eating a nutrient-dense diet rich in whole grains, fruits, vegetables, healthy fats, and fish, while limiting saturated fat (no more than 10 percent of total daily calories), added sugars (no more than 10 percent of total calories), sodium (no more than 2,300 milligrams per day), and limiting alcoholic beverages (if consumed) to two drinks or less a day for men and one drink or less for women. Specifically, it suggests that Americans adopt one of three healthful diet patterns:

▶ **The "Healthy U.S.-Style Pattern,"** which includes whole grains, fruits, vegetables, low-fat dairy, lean protein, eggs, and healthy fats;

- The "Healthy Vegetarian Pattern," which includes whole grains, fruits, vegetables, soyfoods, legumes, nuts, seeds, and healthy fats; and
- The "Healthy Mediterranean-Style Pattern," which includes fish, whole grains, fruits, vegetables, low-fat dairy, olive oil, nuts, and seeds.

The DASH diet (Dietary Approaches to Stop Hypertension), which is the basis for the Healthy U.S.-Style Pattern recommended in the *Dietary Guidelines for Americans,* emphasizes whole plant foods, lean proteins, and low-fat or nonfat dairy foods. The health benefits of vegetarian and vegan eating patterns, such as lower risks of cardiovascular disease, obesity, type 2 diabetes, and certain types of cancer, have been confirmed repeatedly by rigorous studies. The Mediterranean-style diet, a plant-based, whole-foods diet with fish as the primary animal protein and olive oil as the main source of added fat, has been linked with multiple benefits in thousands of studies, including healthy aging, lower risks of chronic diseases, and better cognitive performance. In one study, older adults who followed a Mediterranean-style diet performed better on tests that assessed cognitive functions such as memory and verbal ability. And newer research suggests additional brain benefits can be gained by "going green" with the Mediterranean diet (see "'Green' Mediterranean Diet May Protect the Aging Brain").

What do all of these healthful dietary patterns have in common? They emphasize whole, minimally processed, nutrient-rich foods, such as whole grains, pulses, fruits, vegetables, nuts, seeds, fish, herbs, and spices. When you consume these foods, you are rewarded with a host of essential nutrients, such as vitamins, minerals, fiber, and other compounds that offer health benefits. These foods pack a big nutrition punch for a moderate number of calories.

Another dietary pattern called the MIND diet (Mediterranean-DASH Intervention for Neurodegenerative Delay) has been linked with a reduced risk of dementia. The MIND diet combines two proven healthy diets—the Mediterranean-style and DASH diets—and emphasizes specific foods in each that are associated with better brain health and a lower risk of cognitive decline. The MIND diet includes at least six servings per week of green leafy vegetables, two or more servings per week of berries, olive oil as the primary cooking oil, nuts instead of processed snacks, fish once a week, and getting most proteins from plant sources.

The Power of Plant Foods

Every whole, edible plant contains phytochemicals, compounds that help protect them from environmental threats such as sun damage, insects, pests, and viruses. These compounds are what give plants their distinctive colors and/or flavors, such as the vivid green colors of spinach and avocados, the bright orange hue of carrots and mangos, the spicy bite of chili peppers, and the distinctive aromas of onions and garlic. Scientists have identified thousands of phytochemicals in plant foods, and more continue to be discovered.

In addition to protecting plant foods, phytochemicals help protect people who consume these foods. Research has revealed that phytochemicals have anti-inflammatory and antioxidant properties that help prevent the oxidative stress and chronic inflammation that contribute to many chronic diseases. Other health benefits associated with phytochemicals include destroying cancer cells, repairing DNA damage, and detoxifying carcinogens (cancer-causing substances).

Some phytochemicals have been linked with specific health benefits. For example, a carotenoid called lycopene—the compound that gives tomatoes,

NEW FINDING

"Green" Mediterranean Diet May Protect the Aging Brain

The "green-Med" diet—a Mediterranean-style diet enhanced with green foods high in polyphenols—may help protect against brain atrophy (shrinkage), according to a study conducted in Israel. The researchers divided 284 participants into three groups that followed a healthy diet, a Mediterranean diet, or a "green" Mediterranean diet, which included three to four cups of green tea daily and a shake made of Mankai, a type of aquatic plant with a high polyphenol content. All of the diets also were low in red and processed meats. When researchers reviewed the participants' brain MRIs taken before and after the diets were followed, they found less age-related brain atrophy among those who adhered to either form of the Mediterranean diet, with the least atrophy observed among the "green-Med" diet group. The least atrophy was seen in the brains of participants over age 50. The researchers suggested the benefits of the green-Med diet were due to its high content of polyphenols, micronutrients that are especially high in green plant foods.

The American Journal of Clinical Nutrition, May 2022

Cocoa Flavanols May Reduce Risk for Cardiovascular Death

Participants in the Cocoa Supplement and Multivitamin Outcomes Study (COSMOS) trial included more than 21,000 adults ages 60 and older in the U.S. The participants were randomly assigned to consume cocoa extract containing 500 milligrams of flavanols or a placebo daily. During a median follow-up period of 3.6 years, cocoa flavanol consumption was associated with a 27 percent lower incidence of cardiovascular deaths, but not with a reduction in total cardiovascular events. Additional studies are needed to gain a greater understanding of the potential cardiovascular benefits of cocoa flavanol.

American Journal of Clinical Nutrition, March 2022

Plant-Based Diet May Protect Against Cognitive Decline

Data have indicated that Black people are nearly twice as likely to develop dementia as non-Hispanic white people, but choosing to follow a predominantly plant-based diet may help reduce this risk. To evaluate the relationship between a plant-based diet and the rate of cognitive decline, researchers gathered diet quality data from 4,753 participants (average age 74 years, 62 percent Black, 63 percent female). Black participants whose diets were highest in whole plant foods, such as whole grains, beans, nuts, vegetables, and fruits, had a slower rate of decline in overall cognition, perceptual speed, and episodic memory than Black participants whose diets contained more processed foods with refined grains and added sugars or more animal fat from foods such as meat, dairy, and eggs. The white study participants who followed diets highest in plant-based foods also had a slower rate of cognitive decline, but not to the same degree as the Black participants who followed similar diets.

American Heart Association. Scientific Sessions, March 2022

watermelon, and red bell peppers their red color—is associated with a lower risk of prostate cancer. Isothiocyanates, which are found in cruciferous vegetables such as broccoli, cauliflower, and cabbage, have been linked with protection against heart disease, cancer, and neurodegenerative conditions. Consuming more flavonoids—a large group of phytochemicals that includes flavonols, isoflavones, and anthocyanins—has been linked with healthful aging and a reduced risk of chronic diseases, including cardiovascular disease (see "Cocoa Flavanols May Reduce Risk for Cardiovascular Death"). A previous study also indicated that consuming more flavanol-rich foods (like tea, berries, apples, and cocoa) may help reduce blood pressure. And other research has linked diets higher in phytochemicals with better brain function in older adults.

The more varieties of colorful plant foods you eat, the greater number of phytochemicals you'll get—one of the reasons why it's wise to include a "rainbow" of whole plant foods in your dietary pattern.

Focus on Whole Foods

Eating more plant foods is a good idea, but keep in mind that not all plant foods are created equal. Whole, unrefined foods, like blackberries, walnuts, mushrooms, kale, lentils, and quinoa, are higher in phytochemicals and other valuable nutrients than highly processed foods, especially food products that are high in refined flour and/or added sugar, such as pastries, cookies, sugary sodas, and many varieties of bread, rolls, bagels, and crackers.

While it's true that some processed foods, such as nutrition bars and veggie chips, are technically "plant foods," their nutrient content is usually much lower than whole foods. For example, when whole grains are processed, they are broken down and stripped of their nutritious outer coverings, which reduces their nutritional value. Often, they are then mixed with less healthful ingredients, such as salt, sugar, and saturated fat. Basically, the more a food is altered, the more highly processed it is—and the fewer nutrients it contains.

It's not surprising that research shows some plant-based diets are healthier than others (see "Plant-Based Diet May Protect Against Cognitive Decline"). Diets that are high in refined, highly processed foods do not provide the same health benefits as those that are based on whole or minimally processed plant foods; in fact, they may raise the risk of certain health problems (see "Ultra-processed Foods Linked to Inflammatory Bowel Disease").

It's also important to distinguish between minimally processed and highly processed foods. Many foods must go through some degree of processing to make it to the supermarket; for example, lots of fruits and vegetables are washed and packaged before arriving in the produce section. However, during this type of processing, the food itself remains intact. Minimally processed foods also include whole foods like fruits, vegetables, and beans that have been canned, frozen, or cooked without added sugar or salt. Many of these foods provide as much or more nutrients than their fresh counterparts.

Keeping canned and frozen foods on hand helps ensure that you always have nutrient-rich foods available, regardless of what is currently in season. They're also affordable, convenient, and cut meal prep time. These items also can be more environmentally friendly choices than out-of-season fresh produce, which may travel hundreds or thousands of miles to get to your plate, and often loses some nutrients in the process.

The Story on Supplements

Many people wonder if they need to take vitamin and mineral supplements to boost their health. Taking supplements can help fill some nutrient gaps and deficiencies in your diet, but nutrients in pill form will never measure up to whole plant foods, which are packed with a synergistic array of phytochemicals, fiber, vitamins, and minerals in every bite. That's why studies consistently find health benefits related to eating *whole* foods, but not to *isolated* nutrients obtained from supplements. Also, following a dietary pattern that provides a consistent variety of whole foods means that you'll be less likely to have any significant nutrient deficiencies.

Another advantage of getting nutrients from foods is that they are found in an ideal balance. It's difficult to get too much of a particular nutrient from a diet rich in whole foods, but it's possible to overdo it when you take nutrients in pill form. Some supplements can cause health problems if you take too much, and they may have potentially harmful interactions with medications. And since supplements are not regulated by the U.S. Food & Drug Administration, they may contain more or less of the nutrients and other ingredients that appear on the label, as well as potentially harmful substances, such as heavy metals, that do not appear on the label.

That said, in some cases, physicians do recommend taking supplements to correct deficiencies. Older adults are at increased risk of deficiencies in certain nutrients, such as vitamin D, which plays an essential role in keeping bones strong and reducing fracture risk. Reasons for D deficiency include a decreased ability to synthesize the most active form of D from sunlight and insufficient exposure to sunlight. Certain medical conditions like celiac disease and inflammatory bowel disease, as well as several types of medication, can cause reduced absorption of vitamin D (and many other nutrients). And food sources of vitamin D are limited, so it can be difficult to get enough D from your diet.

If you think you may not be getting enough vitamin D or other nutrients, ask your doctor if you should have a blood test that measures the vitamin D level in your blood. If you are low in D and your doctor advises taking vitamin D supplements, follow his or her recommendations regarding the potency and dosage that you need.

Choose "Super" Foods

For optimal health, choose an eating pattern based on a diverse range of minimally processed "super" plant foods—vegetables, fruits, whole grains, pulses, nuts, and seeds—along with seafood. Due to their superior nutritional content, these "superfoods" offer health benefits beyond the basics of furnishing the substances your body needs to function.

Include several superfoods in your meal plan each day. In the last section of this book, you'll find recipes that feature superfoods from every category: proteins, whole grains, vegetables, fruits, beverages, and flavorful additions, such as fats and spices. But don't lose sight of your overall dietary pattern; adding a few superfoods to your diet won't be of much benefit if the majority of your diet consists of highly processed, low-nutrient food products. Keep in mind that it's your *total* diet that counts in the long run.

NEW FINDING

Ultraprocessed Foods Linked to Inflammatory Bowel Disease

Researchers from the multinational PURE (Prospective Urban Rural Epidemiology) cohort study identified an association between intake of ultraprocessed foods and the risk of developing inflammatory bowel disease (IBD). More than 116,000 adult participants from various geographical regions around the world completed food frequency questionnaires. Researchers analyzed the dietary data they collected to document intake patterns of ultraprocessed foods; they tracked the participants at least every three years over a median of 9.7 years. The researchers found that consuming one or more servings of ultraprocessed foods per day was related to a higher risk of developing incident IBD compared to those consuming one serving or less per day.

The BMJ, July 15, 2021

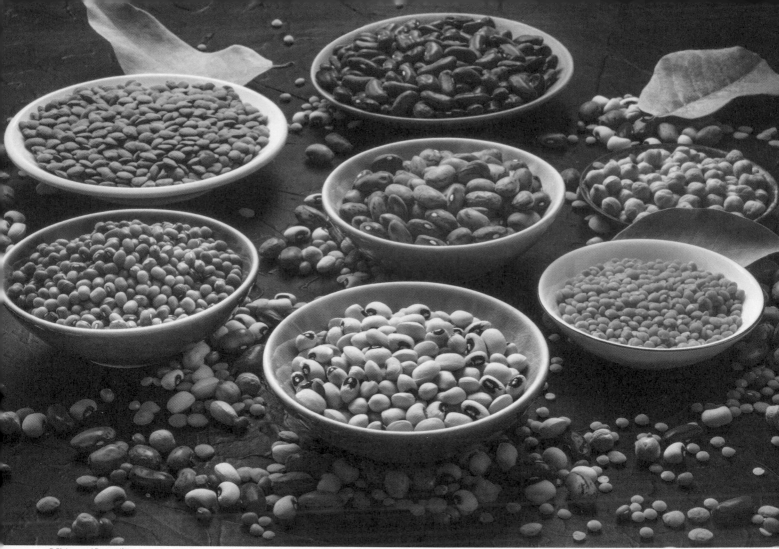

Protein provides the building blocks for structures and substances throughout your body, including bones, blood, muscles, hormones, and enzymes.

2 Proteins

Dietary protein plays a major role in many essential functions throughout your body. In fact, every cell in your body contains some protein. The body utilizes protein and the material it provides to support the development and repair of muscles, bone, blood, and skin. Additionally, protein is required for a healthy immune system and for proper kidney function. And protein contributes to the formation of many important substances, including hormones, neurotransmitters, and enzymes.

Once you consume protein, it is broken down into amino acids, which your body uses as building blocks to create new proteins that have specific functions. For example, hemoglobin is a protein that carries oxygen in the bloodstream. There are 20 types of amino acids that serve as

building blocks; nine of them are called "essential" amino acids because they can only be obtained from food. (The other 11 are made by your body.)

Proteins from animal sources (meat, poultry, fish, and dairy products) are often referred to as "complete" or "high-quality" proteins, because they typically contain all of the essential amino acids. The majority of protein-rich plant foods lack one or more of the essential amino acids, so they are sometimes called "incomplete" proteins. (The plant foods that contain all nine essential amino acids include quinoa, buckwheat, and soybeans.) However, this doesn't mean you can't get the amino acids you need from plant foods; it simply means that at least a few different protein-rich plant foods need to be consumed throughout the day to get them. Also, your body doesn't store protein, but amino acids must be replenished continually, so it's important to include protein in most, if not all, meals and snacks.

Common food pairings that provide all of the essential amino acids are beans and rice, hummus and pita bread, and peanut butter and crackers. Other advantages of plant proteins are that they are higher in fiber, lower in saturated fat, less expensive, and friendlier to the climate and environment than most animal proteins.

Your Protein Needs

The National Academy of Medicine recommends a daily minimum of 0.8 grams of protein per kilogram of body weight, or just over 7 grams for every 20 pounds of body weight for adults. For a person that weighs 150 pounds, that's about 55 grams of protein per day. (As a reference, two large whole eggs provide 12 grams of protein, a 3-ounce serving of meat, fish, or poultry provides about 21 grams, one cup of milk provides 8 grams, and two tablespoons of peanut butter provides 7 grams.)

Other research suggests that more protein—about 10 grams per 20 pounds—may be better for building and sustaining muscle mass, especially for older adults. In this instance, a 150-pound person would need 68 to 82 grams of protein per day, and a 200-pound person would need 91 to 109 grams of protein per day.

These numbers are approximate recommendations, and most people don't need to keep a tally of the grams of protein they consume. In general, you'll get adequate protein if you include a protein-rich food source—pulses (lentils, peas, and beans, including soybeans), low-fat dairy, poultry, fish, nuts, and seeds—with each meal and snack. Also, keep in mind that the overall quality of the protein foods you choose is as important as the amount of protein you eat.

The Protein Package

There's more to protein foods than the grams of protein they contain. When choosing protein foods, consider the complete package—the other substances and nutrients in addition to protein, such as saturated fat, fiber, vitamins, and minerals—that are found in each protein-rich food. It's what's in the total protein package that has led nutrition experts to recommend eating more plant-sourced proteins and fewer animal-sourced proteins (see "Less Meat Consumption Tied to Lower Cancer Risk").

Some animal-sourced protein foods are high in saturated fat and cholesterol, which have been linked with various health risks in hundreds of clinical studies. For example, eating a diet that's high in red meat (beef, veal, pork, mutton, lamb, and goat) is associated with increased risks of mortality (death), heart disease, type 2 diabetes, and kidney disease. One study found that people who consumed meat three or more times per week had more adverse health events than those who ate meat less often. Other research suggests that dietary patterns lower in red meat are linked with a lower risk of colon cancer. The American Institute for Cancer Research (AICR) and the International Agency for Research on Cancer (IARC) recommend limiting red meat to no more than three portions per week.

An even greater concern is processed meat—meat that has been altered to enhance the flavor or preserve the food. Common processing methods include salting, smoking, curing, and fermentation. Processed meats, such as sausage, bacon, hot dogs, ham, pepperoni, and salami, are often very high in sodium and saturated fat. The IARC has classified processed meat as "carcinogenic to humans," one of the only foods to earn this classification. The IARC announced this after a group of scientists reviewed more than 800 studies and found

Less Meat Consumption Tied to Lower Cancer Risk

Diets higher in plant foods and lower in meat have been linked with a lower risk of cancer, according to a study conducted in the United Kingdom. The 472,377 participants were cancer-free at the study's outset and were followed for an average of 11.4 years. The participants were grouped according to dietary practices: regular meat-eaters who consumed processed meat, red meat (beef, lamb, mutton, or pork), or poultry more than five times per week; low meat-eaters who consumed processed meat, red meat, or poultry five or fewer times per week; fish-eaters who never consumed red meat, processed meat, or poultry; and vegetarian. The researchers found that, compared with regular meat-eaters, people who were low meat-eaters, fish-eaters, or vegetarian had lower risks of all types of cancer. Men who were low meat-eaters had a lower risk of colorectal cancer, and men who were fish-eaters or vegetarian had lower risks of prostate cancer. Postmenopausal women following vegetarian diet patterns had lower risks of breast cancer.

BMC Medicine, February 2022

conclusive evidence that regular consumption of processed meat increases the risk of colorectal and stomach cancers. The AICR and the IARC recommend avoiding processed meat altogether.

Fortunately, many protein sources come in a healthier package. For example, along with protein, seafood provides vitamin D and omega-3 fatty acids, nutrients with cardioprotective benefits that may reduce the risk of neurodegenerative diseases and boost the immune system. Fatty fish, such as salmon, sardines, mackerel, and herring, are highest in omega-3s, and are a key food group in many beneficial dietary patterns, such as the traditional Mediterranean-style diet.

Plant sources of protein, such as soy, lentils, peas, beans, nuts, and seeds, offer a healthy package of bonus nutrients, including fiber, vitamins, minerals, phytochemicals, and healthy fats, along with protein. In fact, many studies have shown that, by adopting a plant-based dietary pattern, which includes eating more plant proteins and fewer animal proteins, you can lower your risks of chronic diseases, such as heart disease, cancer, and type 2 diabetes, as well as extend your life. One Harvard study estimated that early death rates could be decreased by 10 percent by increasing consumption of plant-based foods.

To reduce the animal-sourced foods in your diet, start including a few meatless meals featuring plant proteins, like a simple stir-fry with tofu or a veggie burrito filled with black beans, in your weekly meal plan. You can also consider switching to a vegetarian or vegan diet for added health benefits. Another benefit of a diet high in plant protein is a reduced impact on the planet; several studies have rated vegetarian and vegan diet patterns best for reducing your environmental footprint.

The most healthful protein choices include seafood, soyfoods (edamame, tofu, tempeh, and soymilk), pulses (beans, lentils, and peas), seeds, nuts, skinless poultry, and low-fat dairy. We highlight some of these protein-rich foods on our superfoods list due to their excellent nutritional profiles and research-based benefits.

Fatty Fish

If you consume animal foods, aim to put fish on your plate a couple of times per week. Seafood is an excellent source of protein, and it's lower in calories and much lower in saturated fat than many other animal foods, such as beef and pork. Don't let the word "fatty" frighten you; most of the fat found in cold-water fatty fish is in the form of unsaturated fat, such as omega-3 fatty acids, which have been linked with beneficial properties.

Fatty fish, which includes salmon, herring, sardines, and mackerel, is the primary source of the omega-3 fatty acids docosahexaenoic acid (DHA) and eicosapentaenoic acid (EPA) in our diets. These fats are good for your heart whether you do or don't have heart disease. Eating omega-3-rich fish can lower your risk of arrhythmias (irregular heartbeats), reduce levels of triglycerides and blood pressure, and slow the growth of plaque in your arteries. In addition, consuming omega-3s may yield other advantages, such as protection from inflammation, arthritis, depression, diabetes, Alzheimer's disease, and colorectal cancer.

Both the American Heart Association and the 2020–2025 *Dietary Guidelines for Americans* recommend consuming two 4-ounce servings of fish per week. And the Healthy Mediterranean-Style Diet suggests eating 15 ounces of fish, or about four servings, each week. Try serving baked flounder or snapper with whole-wheat pasta and vegetables, grilled salmon with lemon and dill, or blackened tilapia or shrimp in tacos.

Also be aware that scientists are increasingly concerned about the global fish supply. Many fish species are threatened due to overfishing, and destructive fishing methods can have long-lasting effects on our oceans. In addition, fish are exposed to environmental contaminants, such as mercury, polychlorinated biphenyls (PCBs), and dioxins.

One way to help alleviate the strain on the global fish supply is to be selective about your fish choices. The top environmentally friendly fish choices include albacore tuna (troll, pole, and line-caught), Pacific cod, shrimp (U.S. farmed), and New Zealand salmon, according to the Monterey Bay Aquarium. Download the organization's Seafood Watch app (seafoodwatch.org), or ask your fishmonger, farmers market vendor, or restaurant professional for the best choices in your region.

Finally, limit your consumption of the fish with the highest mercury content, which includes the following, according to the National Resources Defense Council: orange roughy, tuna (ahi and bigeye), king mackerel, marlin, shark, swordfish, and tilefish (from the Gulf of Mexico).

Pulses

Pulses, which include beans, lentils, and peas, are the mature seeds of flowering plants, and are part of a broader category of plant foods called legumes.

Pulses have served as a cornerstone for traditional diets around the globe for centuries, from pinto beans in Central America to chickpeas in the Middle East. In fact, they are one of a trio of foods found in the pre-Columbian agricultural tradition known as "The Three Sisters"; beans were planted at the base of maize (corn), along with squash. This companion planting provided nitrogen and moisture for the soil, and the maize offered a natural "trellis" for the bean vines to climb. These three historic "superfoods" were key sources of nutrition in original dietary patterns.

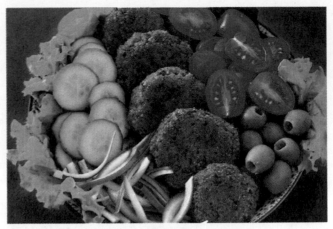

For a meatless meal that's high in protein, try falafel, a Middle-Eastern vegetarian dish made with chickpeas and spices.

© Gauravmasand | Dreamstime

Pulses are versatile, easy to prepare, shelf-stable (in dried or canned form), sustainable (they get nitrogen from the air and "fix" it in the soil, so they don't need nitrogen-based fertilizers to thrive), and economical. These plant foods offer an array of nutrients, including fiber, folate, manganese, potassium, iron, magnesium, copper, selenium, and zinc, in addition to protein. Like other plant foods, pulses contain phytochemicals with anti-inflammatory properties.

Consuming fiber in foods, including pulses, has been linked with lowering blood cholesterol levels and inflammation, reducing weight, and reducing the risk of heart disease, hypertension, diabetes, and some types of cancer. In fact, a 2020 study reported an 8 percent lower incidence of breast cancer in women consuming the highest amount of dietary fiber compared to women consuming the least amount of fiber.

Pulses are easy to fit into your eating plan. Soak dried beans in water overnight, drain the water, add fresh water or broth, and cook them up with your favorite seasonings and vegetables. A slow cooker or Instant Pot can make this even easier.

Cook up a pot of lentils to serve with whole grains like brown rice, bulgur wheat, or quinoa for a budget-friendly, satisfying meal. Blend chickpeas with olive oil, lemon juice, garlic, and tahini into homemade hummus (a great dip

Protein-Rich Pulses

- Adzuki beans
- Black beans
- Black-eyed peas (cow peas)
- Cannellini beans
- Chickpeas (garbanzo beans)
- Cranberry beans
- Fava beans
- Great Northern beans
- Kidney beans
- Lima beans
- Mung beans
- Navy beans
- Pinto beans
- Small red beans
- Lentils (black, green, red, yellow)
- Split peas

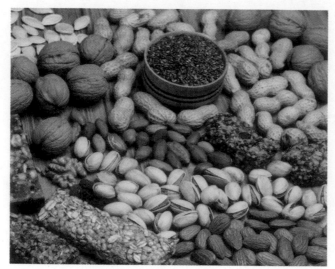

for vegetables or a sandwich spread), or mash cooked beans and combine them with oats and shredded or diced veggies to make meatless burgers.

Canned beans are an easy, economical choice. Look for canned beans with no added salt, or rinse and drain the beans to reduce levels of sodium by up to 41 percent. Or if you prefer to make bean dishes "from scratch," keep a few bags of dried beans on hand in your pantry. Natural and specialty food stores may offer an even wider selection, especially in bulk bins. Look for heritage or heirloom beans, which are unique varieties of beans with different colors, texture, and flavors that farmers have treasured through the centuries.

Nuts

Hundreds of studies have documented a number of health benefits linked to nut consumption. And there's no need to steer clear of nuts because of their fat content: The majority of the fat in nuts is healthy, unsaturated fat, which has been linked with providing protection against cardiovascular disease, diabetes, and some cancers. Including nuts in your diet may even help prevent obesity, as recent studies show that people who eat nuts tend to gain less weight than people who rarely eat them. While *all* nuts are good for you,

including almonds, walnuts, pistachios, pine nuts, cashews, macadamias, Brazil nuts, pecans, hazelnuts, and peanuts (which actually are legumes, but are nutritionally similar to nuts), we focus on a few that boast particularly powerful nutrient profiles that give them superfood status.

Walnuts

Including walnuts in a healthy dietary pattern has been shown to reduce the risk of coronary heart disease, which has earned them a qualified health claim from the U.S. Food & Drug Administration. These tree nuts also have been linked to decreased risks of cancer, cognitive decline, type 2 diabetes, obesity, and hypertension, as well as improved fertility and gut health.

Walnuts are rich in fiber, manganese, copper, magnesium, and phosphorus, in addition to 4 grams of protein in a single ounce (about 14 halves). They also contain a variety of phytochemicals with antioxidant and anti-inflammatory properties. In a study of adults in their 60s and 70s, researchers found that consumers of walnuts had lower levels of inflammatory markers that were strongly linked to heart disease than people who did not eat walnuts, suggesting that the anti-inflammatory effects of walnuts may contribute to their heart-protecting ability.

Walnuts are the only nut that contains a significant amount of alpha-linolenic acid (ALA), a form of omega-3 fatty acids found in plant foods. While much of the evidence on omega-3 benefits is based on studies of the long-chain varieties (EPA and DHA) found in fatty fish, the short-chain, ALA has its own anti-inflammatory benefits. Additionally, a small percentage of ALA is converted to EPA and DHA in the body.

It's easy to add walnuts to your dietary pattern: Sprinkle a handful (about one-quarter cup) over cereal or oatmeal, spinach salad, or stir into yogurt or a grain-based dish such as tabouli (a traditional Middle-Eastern dish made with bulgur wheat, parsley, mint, olive oil, lemon juice, and tomatoes). Or combine them with some raisins, dried berries, or apricots for a simple, satisfying snack. You can even use ground walnuts, with their "meaty" texture, in place of ground beef in spaghetti sauce or taco filling.

Peanuts

The peanut is a legume (it grows below the ground in a pod), but it's categorized as a nut due to its nutritional and culinary similarities to tree nuts. These nutrition powerhouses pack 7 grams of protein into each one-ounce serving (about 28 whole nuts)—the highest protein content of all nuts. They are also filled with heart-healthy fats and fiber, and they are particularly high in the amino acid arginine, a precursor to the compound nitric oxide, which helps expand blood vessels. Regular consumption of peanuts also has been linked to a lower stroke risk (see "Eating Peanuts May Help Reduce Risk of Stroke").

Each handful of peanuts provides niacin, thiamin, choline, vitamin E, magnesium, zinc, iron, copper, as well as phytochemicals such as resveratrol, the antioxidant found in red wine. Plus, peanuts are easy on their growing environment, since they have the ability to "fix" nitrogen in the soil, meaning they don't require nitrogen-containing fertilizers that can stimulate the release of carbon dioxide and other harmful greenhouse gases into the air.

Munching on one ounce (about one-quarter cup) of peanuts daily has been linked with numerous health benefits, such as a reduced risk of chronic diseases, lower blood lipids and inflammation levels, and better weight management. Peanuts contain a nutrient trifecta of protein, fat, and fiber that helps control hunger. Enjoy the classic flavor and texture of peanut butter on whole-grain toast, with fruit or veggie slices, in smoothies, or in a tasty sauce for Asian noodle dishes. Skip brands that contain added sugar and/or oil and stick with brands that contain only peanuts. Chances are, at least a few food stores in your area sell freshly ground peanut butter and/or provide the machine and the nuts so you can grind your own.

Almonds

Almonds are high in healthy, monounsaturated fat and rich in protein, providing 6 grams per ounce (about 24 almonds), which is almost as much as the 7 to 8 grams found in an ounce of meat. Almonds also contain riboflavin (vitamin B$_2$), magnesium, phosphorus, and calcium, and they are a top food source of vitamin E, a powerful antioxidant that has been linked with lower risks of cancer and Alzheimer's disease.

Noshing on almonds brings plenty of benefits supported by a body of scientific research, including better blood cholesterol levels and cardiovascular health, better weight control, and improved blood glucose control for type 2 diabetes patients. It all boils down to their trio of nutrients—fiber, healthy fats, and protein—which help promote a sense of fullness. Like all tree nuts, almonds are calorie-dense (160 calories

NEW FINDING

Eating Peanuts May Help Reduce Risk of Stroke

Including peanuts in your diet may help decrease stroke risk, according to Japanese researchers. A total of 74,793 Japanese study participants ages 45 to 74 years old were followed for a median of 14.8 years. Food frequency questionnaires were utilized to collect dietary data that included the participants' peanut consumption. The study participants who consumed the most peanuts had a 16 percent lower risk of total stroke, a 20 percent lower risk of ischemic stroke (the most common type of stroke, usually caused by a blood clot blocking a blood vessel and cutting off blood flow to the brain), and a 13 percent lower risk of cardiovascular disease than the participants who consumed no peanuts. These health benefits may, in part, be due to the high content of unsaturated fats in peanuts, along with other nutrients such as magnesium, vitamin E, and dietary fiber.

Stroke, Sept. 9, 2021

in one ounce), but research shows that they (and other nuts) may provide up to 20 percent fewer calories than previously thought, because the fiber in nuts may decrease calorie absorption.

There are countless ways to include almonds in your diet. Enjoy them as is for a quick and satisfying snack, add slivered almonds to green salads and vegetable dishes, stir them into muffins and pancake batters, and use ground almonds as a breading for baked fish or a casserole topping.

Pistachios

Pistachios provide a good dose of protein, healthy unsaturated fats, fiber, and B vitamins in every one-ounce serving (49 nuts). Pistachios have the highest potassium content among all varieties of nuts. In addition, they contain magnesium, copper, zinc, iron, and phytochemicals, including carotenoids, which impart that lovely shade of green.

Research has linked pistachio consumption with several health benefits, such as controlling glucose and cholesterol levels. Eating pistachios may even aid in weight management, especially if you shell them yourself; research has shown that you gain a greater sense of satiety by opening the shell and eating the nut than by simply tossing already shelled pistachios into your mouth.

To go beyond simple snacking, try adding pistachios to homemade granola, vegetable salads, and grain pilafs, or grind them into a "butter" and use as a spread for whole-grain toast or crackers. For a fresh take on pesto (usually made with pine nuts), blend pistachios with some olive oil, garlic, basil or parsley, and a bit of Parmesan, and toss with whole-grain pasta.

Seeds

Seeds are perfect examples of nutritional powerhouses that come in small packages. Seeds, which are essentially the tiny embryos of plants, are rich in healthful nutrients, including protein, healthy fats, fiber, vitamins, minerals, and phytochemicals. There are many types of edible seeds around the world, but the most common include flax, pumpkin, sunflower, sesame, chia, and hemp. All of these seeds are worth including in your diet, but we're focusing on a few super seeds that are the cream of the crop, nutritionally speaking.

Flaxseed

Flax has been grown in the Mediterranean region for thousands of years. Flax has been put to use in a number of ways, yielding material for fabric, string, and linseed oil for wood preservation. The seeds of the flax plant contain a number of valuable nutrients, including heart-healthy unsaturated fats, ALA (a plant-based omega-3 fatty acid), a compound called lignan that has powerful antioxidant action, and mucilage, a gel-forming fiber that improves absorption of nutrients. Every one-ounce serving of flaxseed (about three tablespoons) offers 5 grams of protein, 8 grams of dietary fiber, and thiamin, magnesium, zinc, calcium, iron, copper, and manganese.

With all of those healthful nutrients, it's no surprise that eating flaxseed has been linked with decreasing LDL cholesterol and blood pressure levels, plaque buildup in arteries, and risk of cancer, while improving blood glucose levels and easing constipation.

Those tiny brown seeds are bursting with versatility. Add them to your morning smoothie, mix them into homemade veggie balls (ground flaxseed will help provide thickening without the need for eggs), sprinkle them over your yogurt or cereal, and stir them into batters and doughs for baked goods such as muffins and breads. Keep in mind that whole flaxseed isn't broken down in your digestive tract, so you'll need to consume ground flaxseed (you can grind it yourself or purchase it already ground, in which case it may be called flax meal) to reap the benefits inside those tiny but tough outer hulls.

Chia Seeds

In recent years, chia seeds have garnered mainstream attention, but these small black seeds aren't new—they were important dietary staples of the Mayans, Aztecs, Incans, and Native Americans centuries ago.

Chia seeds provide a healthy dose of protein (4 grams) in a one-ounce serving (about two tablespoons), as well as plant-based omega-3 fatty acids in the form of ALA. And, with 11 grams of fiber per serving, chia seeds are the top fiber providers among seed varieties, so they can help you feel full longer. Chia seeds also are rich in key minerals, including calcium, phosphorus, manganese, and iron.

One unique feature of chia seeds is their ability to form a gel when combined with water or other liquids. This action can help bind ingredients together, so chia can be used as a replacement for eggs in many recipes, such as muffins, pancakes, and waffles. A general rule of thumb is to mix one tablespoon of chia seeds with three tablespoons of water and substitute it for one egg in a recipe. Let the seeds soak for about 10 minutes to gel.

Chia seeds have a mild, nutty flavor that goes well with a variety of foods and beverages, both sweet and savory. Mix chia seeds with lemon or lime juice and water to make a beverage called chia fresca, and combine with water, fruit juice, milk, or plant-based beverages to create a pudding-like consistency. Chia seeds can also serve as a binder in savory dishes, such as salmon or crab cakes and bean- or lentil-based veggie patties.

Hemp Seeds

The hemp seed is a treasure trove of nutrients, versatility, and taste. Hemp and marijuana are both members of the cannabis plant group, but hemp has an extremely low tetrahydrocannabinol (THC) content (the substance that gives marijuana its psychoactive properties) and does not cause a "high" when ingested.

Hemp seeds have an impressive nutrient profile: 10 grams of protein and 10 grams of heart-healthy omega-3 and omega-6 fats per ounce (about three tablespoons), along with iron, thiamin, magnesium, zinc, manganese, various phytochemicals, and 3 grams of fiber. Although research on hemp seeds is limited, thus far, studies have linked them with reduced risks of cardiovascular disease, obesity, and type 2 diabetes.

Hemp seeds (also called hemp hearts) are surging in popularity among farmers as a sustainable food source, and they are excellent in many ways in the kitchen. They will add valuable protein to breakfast porridge, pasta dishes, smoothies, and fruit or veggie salads. You also can use culinary hemp oil and hemp butter in recipes as a nutritious substitute for other nut and seed oils and butters.

Sunflower Seeds

Inside the large head of the mature sunflower is an artistic spiral of hundreds of nutritious seeds. A one-ounce serving (about three tablespoons) of shelled sunflower seeds provides more than one-third of the daily recommended amount of vitamin E, a powerful antioxidant vitamin that many people fall short on. In addition, sunflower seeds are rich in copper, niacin, manganese, selenium, zinc, folate, and pantothenic acid, as well as heart-healthy fats, protein (5 grams per ounce), fiber (3 grams per ounce), and phytochemicals, such as cholesterol-lowering phytosterols.

Since nature packages sunflower seeds in hard, thick shells, you can turn to these seeds as on-the-go nutrition,

Protein in Soy Foods		
FOOD	SERVING SIZE	PROTEIN
Edamame (green soybeans), cooked	½ cup	17 g
Soybeans, cooked	½ cup	15 g
Tempeh	½ cup	15 g
Tofu, extra-firm, firm, soft, silken, or baked	½ cup	6–20 g
Soymilk	1 cup	5–9 g
Soynuts	1½ Tbsp	5 g

packing them in gym bags, backpacks, lunchboxes, and purses. These seeds are excellent additions to granola, banana bread, slaws, and pasta dishes. Try sunflower seed butter as a delicious spread on whole-grain toast and as a substitute for butter or margarine in snack bar recipes. Sunflower seed butter can also be thinned with water to create a tasty dressing that can be drizzled over power bowls or salads or used as a dip for falafel, fresh fruit slices, or carrot and celery sticks.

Soy

One of the most nutritious, thoroughly researched foods on the planet is the humble soybean. Soy is rich in plant protein, and unlike most plant proteins, it provides all nine of the essential amino acids. Soybeans are also a great source of fiber and iron, as well as calcium, manganese, potassium, magnesium, copper, and vitamin B_2.

Soybeans also contain various phytochemicals, the most notable of which are isoflavones. Isoflavones are phytoestrogens, plant estrogens that possess antifungal, antimicrobial, and antioxidant properties that help the plant survive;

these protective effects may extend to humans who consume them.

A body of research has linked eating soy to a number of health benefits, including reducing cholesterol levels, lowering the risks of heart disease and prostate cancer, and reducing the frequency of hot flashes experienced by menopausal women.

Despite soy's beneficial nutrients, at one time, there were concerns that it might contribute to estrogen-sensitive breast cancer. However, numerous studies have shown that moderate soy intake poses no increase in breast cancer risk, even for breast cancer survivors, and may even lower the risk of breast cancer and breast cancer recurrence. Research also has shown that Asian populations, who consume large amounts of soy in their traditional dietary patterns, have a lower incidence of breast cancer than populations who consume fewer soyfoods.

Both the American Institute for Cancer Research and the American Cancer Society report that moderate amounts of soyfoods—one to three servings per day—are safe to consume and pose no potential harms to health. The *2020-2025 Dietary Guidelines for Americans* includes soyfoods in two of its recommended healthy eating patterns: the Healthy U.S.-Style and Healthy Vegetarian diets.

To fully enjoy the benefits of soy, choose minimally processed foods made with soybeans, such as edamame (green soybeans, which are often steamed and served in the pod at Japanese and Thai restaurants), tempeh (a fermented soy and grain food originating in Indonesia), tofu, soymilk, and soy nuts. Isolated soy ingredients or supplements do not provide the same nutrients found in whole soy, and the various compounds found in whole soy may be more or less concentrated or absent altogether in supplements.

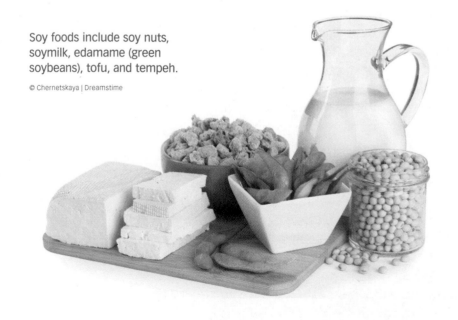

Soy foods include soy nuts, soymilk, edamame (green soybeans), tofu, and tempeh.

© Chernetskaya | Dreamstime

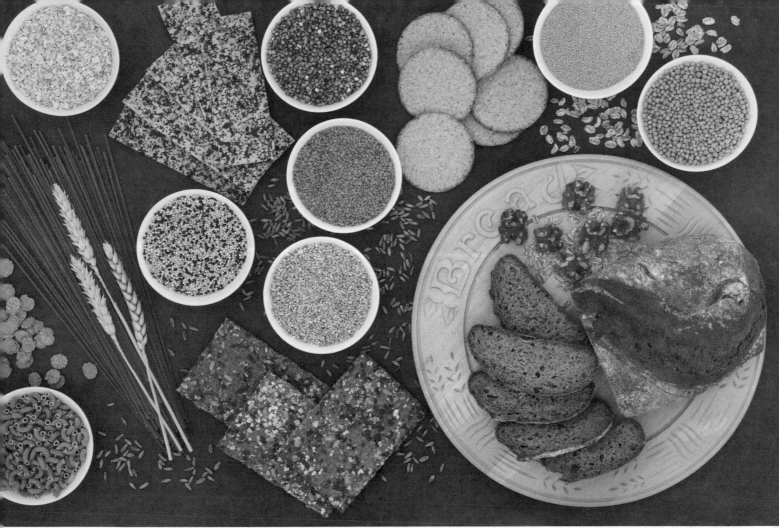

Whole grains are much higher in many nutrients, including fiber, than refined grains.

3 Whole Grains

Grain foods include any food that is produced from wheat, rice, barley, oats, or other cereal grain. When shopping at the local grocery, you'll find a wide variety of grain foods in the shape of breads, tortillas, cereal, rice blends, crackers, and more. The key to getting maximum nutrition from grain-based foods is selecting whole grains rather than refined grains. Whole-grain foods contain the entire grain kernel (bran, germ, and endosperm), and with it, the grain's nutritional potency. Refined-grain foods have had the bran and germ stripped away; the remaining endosperm is low in nutritional value.

Whole grains are an important part of the diet and contribute nutrients that are essential for health and to help prevent disease. Whole grains provide slow-digesting, nutrient-rich carbohydrates (carbs) that are the primary source of fuel for your body. Whole grains are a good source of dietary fiber, vitamins, minerals, antioxidants, and plant compounds such as polyphenols that may contribute additional beneficial effects. Some whole grains also provide a significant amount of protein. The 2020–2025 *Dietary Guidelines for Americans* recommends that adults eat at least half of their grain foods as whole grains. Standard serving sizes for whole grains include one-half cup of cooked oatmeal, pasta, or rice, one slice of bread, or a cup of dry, ready-to-eat cereal.

Clinical research has revealed the many benefits associated with consuming more whole grains and fewer refined grains. Diets stocked with whole

High Fiber-Diet Linked with Reduced Risk of Dementia

Dietary fiber intake is associated with a range of health benefits, including lower risks of colorectal cancer and cardiovascular disease. Now, it appears a reduced risk of dementia can be added to that list of benefits. The Circulatory Risk in Communities Study included Japanese adults ages 40 to 64 who completed dietary surveys between 1985 and 1999. The researchers tracked study participants for incidents of disabling dementia ("requiring care under the national insurance") from 1999 through 2020. During this time, 670 cases of disabling dementia were reported. Analysis of dietary and medical data revealed the participants with the highest intake of dietary fiber had the lowest risk for developing disabling dementia, and the participants with the least fiber intake had the highest risk. The mechanism through which dietary fiber may decrease dementia risk remains under investigation.

Nutritional Neuroscience, February 2022

grains and dietary fiber have been linked to reduced risks of stroke, type 2 diabetes, heart disease, colorectal cancer, asthma, and dementia (see "High Fiber-Diet Linked with Reduced Risk of Dementia"). Another study found that high blood pressure was less likely to develop in adults who reported consuming whole grains "sometimes" or "always" on dietary questionnaires than in those who reported no consumption of whole grains. Eating whole grains also can help you reach and maintain a healthy weight.

On the other hand, dietary patterns that are high in refined grains and low in whole grains are associated with greater chronic disease risk, including diabetes and cardiovascular disease. A 2021 study of adults from 21 countries found that participants with the highest intake of refined grains (about seven servings a day) had a higher risk of total mortality and major cardiovascular events, including non-fatal heart attack, stroke, or heart failure, than participants with the lowest intake (less than one serving per day of refined grains).

Refined Equals Processed

Historians report that whole grains first entered the human diet with the onset of the first farming practices nearly 10,000 years ago. For the last 3,000 to 4,000 years, humans have depended on grains as a main portion of their overall diet.

The practice of refining grains did not begin until centuries later. During the American Industrial Revolution, a process of milling was invented that used machines to remove the bran and germ from whole grains. This was a significant advancement for food merchants and manufacturers, because the flour made from the remaining grain could be stored for much longer periods without spoiling. The refined grain, mostly in the form of white flour, became a primary ingredient in many commercially prepared foods. Today, the typical Western diet is filled with refined grain products, including breads, bagels, muffins, crackers, snack foods, desserts, and breakfast cereals.

The story of refined grains is an important one as it relates to our health. One of the major side effects of eating too many refined grains is reflected in changes that occur in blood glucose levels. Elevated blood glucose is the hallmark indicator of diabetes. Since foods made with refined flour lack the fiber that slows down the absorption of glucose, they cause a more rapid spike in blood glucose levels, which spurs your pancreas to produce insulin to usher that glucose into your tissues. When large amounts of refined grains are consumed regularly, over time, your body may not produce enough insulin to effectively deal with the excess glucose, or it may not use the insulin properly. Either way, the result is chronically high levels of blood glucose.

If glucose levels remain high over a period of years or decades, eventually, it will cause damage to multiple systems and organs in your body, including your blood vessels, eyes, heart, and nervous system. In addition, refined grains do not have the same satiety value (the ability to make you feel full) as fiber-rich whole grains—especially grains in their whole, intact form, such as cooked barley, brown rice, or oats. You're more likely to be hungrier sooner after eating refined grains than whole grains, which can lead to snacking on unhealthy foods and/or overeating.

In addition, the quick rise followed by quick drop in glucose that occurs after eating refined grains may cause a surge of energy that is often followed by low energy and feelings of fatigue. This energy crash can perpetuate a vicious cycle of energy highs and lows produced by repeated consumption of refined grains.

How to Find Whole Grains

If you're looking to make an impactful change in dietary habits for optimal health, prioritize replacing refined grains with whole grains. The 2020-2025 *Dietary Guidelines for Americans* recommends getting at least half of your grain servings from whole grains, which is three daily servings for the average person.

One serving of whole grains is equivalent to 16 grams (a little more than half an ounce). While it's easy to see if foods are authentic whole grains when you're eating a serving of simple intact grains, such as old-fashioned oats, buckwheat, or brown rice, it can be more difficult to determine if food products, such as breads, cereals, nutrition bars, snack foods, and crackers, are made with whole grains.

Reading the ingredients list is the best way to find whole-grain food products in the grocery store. If the first ingredient on the list is a whole grain (for example, whole-wheat flour, oats, brown rice), the food is a good source of whole grains. But if the first ingredient is enriched wheat flour—which is refined white flour that's had some vitamins and minerals added—it's not a good whole-grain source. (Why the first ingredient? Because ingredients are listed from the highest to the lowest by weight, so the food product contains more of the first ingredient than any of the other ingredients.) Also, foods with shorter ingredient lists may be more healthful than those with a long list, especially if the list contains a lot of added sugars and/or non-food items, such as colors, flavorings, emulsifiers, thickeners, and preservatives.

It's particularly important to check the ingredients list if you see a "Made with Whole Grains" claim on the front of the food package. This claim may lead you to mistakenly believe that all of the grains in the product are whole, when, in fact, the product may be made primarily from refined grains and may contain just a small percentage of whole grains.

While *all* whole grains are nutrient-rich and deserve inclusion in your eating plan, the following whole grains have earned superfoods status due to their exceptional nutrition profiles.

When looking for whole-grain foods, check the ingredients list: Enriched flour is NOT a whole grain.

© Daburke | Dreamstime

Wheat

Wheat is considered the "mother grain" of Western civilization, and it is by far the most prevalent grain in the U.S. food supply: In 2019, the estimated amount of wheat flour consumed per capita was 131 pounds. Sadly, this grain has been under attack in recent years. Part of the reason for this is the growing awareness and prevalence of two health conditions: celiac disease and gluten sensitivity. People with these conditions must avoid foods that contain gluten, which include wheat, rye, barley, and triticale. And going gluten-free has grown in popularity among people who don't have to avoid gluten because they believe that a gluten-free diet is "healthier" than a diet with gluten. However, research does not support the idea that wheat is inherently unhealthy for any reason, and gluten-free foods can contain just as much refined grains, added sugars, sodium, and saturated fat as conventional grain-based products.

The moral of the story is that you don't have to avoid wheat or gluten to

Varieties of Whole Wheat

NAME	DESCRIPTION
Bulgur	Called "Middle Eastern pasta," bulgur is whole wheat kernels that have been boiled, dried, and cracked.
Einkorn	One of the most ancient wheat varieties, it can be used whole or as a whole-grain flour.
Farro	An ancient variety of hard wheat, which was a staple in Roman times.
Kamut	A plump, nutty wheat variety with a rich, chewy taste.
Spelt	This wheat variety was popular in certain parts of Europe during medieval times.
Wheat berries	Intact kernels of whole wheat with a chewy, nutty flavor.
Whole-wheat flour	A fine powder milled from whole wheat kernels. Available in different varieties, such as red wheat, white wheat, winter wheat, hard wheat, and soft wheat.

achieve an optimal diet. What is most important is that you focus on what *type* of wheat products you are choosing. Most of the wheat-based foods in the typical Western diet are processed foods like bagels, pretzels, pastries, crackers, cookies, and muffins made from refined flour. However, the availability of whole-wheat foods has grown exponentially in recent years as more Americans have learned about the many health benefits linked with diets rich in whole grains.

Whole wheat offers a wealth of nutrients: One serving (about one-quarter cup dry or one-half cup cooked) of intact grains contains about 6 grams of protein, 6 grams of fiber, and B vitamins, magnesium, zinc, iron, and selenium. Polyphenols, the phytochemicals found in wheat, have antioxidant and anti-inflammatory effects.

Hundreds of studies have documented the health benefits of consuming whole grains; they include reducing the risk of stroke by 30 to 36 percent, type 2 diabetes by 21 to 30 percent, and heart disease by 25 to 28 percent, as well as better weight control and blood pressure levels. American studies that evaluate diets high in whole grains are based largely on the intake of whole wheat, since it is the most commonly consumed whole grain in the U.S.

The benefits associated with whole wheat may be due mainly to its natural fiber content; research continues to confirm fiber's link with protection against colon cancer, obesity, diabetes, and heart disease, as well as contributing to a healthier, more balanced environment in the gut.

Whole wheat comes in many forms and varieties, such as bulgur, einkorn, farro, kamut, spelt, and wheat berries, all of which can be included in a healthy dietary pattern. You can simmer whole-wheat kernels like wheat berries, farro, bulgur, and freekeh and include them in breakfast porridges, grain bowls, side dishes, stews, casseroles, and veggie burgers. When choosing wheat-based products, select breads, crackers, and pasta made with whole-wheat flour.

Rice

Rice is grown on every continent except Antarctica and is among the three leading food crops (along with wheat and corn) worldwide. This simple plant seed is the most widely consumed grain in Asia, accounting for nearly half of the daily calorie intake for billions of people. In the United States, the average consumption of this gluten-free grain is 26 pounds per person per year.

You're probably familiar with basic rice varieties such as white, brown, and wild rice, but with an estimated 40,000 rice varieties around the world, there are plenty of options to explore. Rice even comes in many colors, such as red, purple, and black—all of which are considered whole grains.

Once the inedible hull is removed from a rice kernel, what remains is brown rice, which is a whole grain. If the rice is milled further and the bran and germ are removed, what remains is white, refined rice. Brown long-grain rice has four times the fiber of white long-grain rice, and it has a higher mineral, vitamin, and phytochemical content. More vibrant colors point to a higher phytochemical content; researchers have found that red, purple, and black rice have higher levels of phytochemicals than brown rice.

One serving (one-quarter cup dry or one-half cup cooked) of brown rice provides more than 15 vitamins and minerals, including manganese, phosphorus, magnesium, zinc, copper, selenium, and several B vitamins, as well as protein (3 grams) and fiber (2 grams).

Benefits linked with whole-grain rice intake include lower risks of diabetes and obesity, as well as healthier cholesterol levels. Research has shown that rice eaters have healthier diets overall, with higher consumption of vegetables, legumes, and fruits and lower consumption of saturated fat and added sugars.

Healthy, delicious global rice dishes include stir-fries from China, curry dishes from India, and red beans and rice from the Caribbean. Modern inventions of rice bowls, topped with innovative combinations of vegetables, beans, dried fruit, nuts, and flavorful seasonings, are a hot and healthy culinary trend worth following.

Oats

The familiar oat grain is a power player in the nutrition world. One beneficial attribute of this grain is that it is almost always consumed in its whole form, with the bran and germ intact.

Steel-cut oats are whole oat kernels (also called groats) sliced once or twice into smaller kernels. Old-fashioned oats have been cut, steamed, and flattened (rolled), which reduces cooking time but preserves all of the nutrients. Quick-cooking oats are cut smaller, rolled thinner, and steamed longer than old-fashioned oats, but they still retain all parts of the original grain.

All forms of whole-grain oats are packed with nutrition: One serving (one-half cup cooked) contains 4 grams of fiber and 7 grams of protein, along with iron, thiamin, manganese, and magnesium. Oats are very high in a type of fiber called beta-glucan, which has been linked to heart health and cancer protection, and oats contain phytochemicals that have antioxidant and anti-inflammatory effects.

When it comes to health benefits, oats are best known for their power to reduce LDL ("bad") cholesterol levels. Eating one serving of oats every day is a healthy habit; it can reduce elevated levels of total cholesterol by as much as 23 percent, according to research. And there's more to oats: They can lower blood pressure and blood glucose levels, promote regular bowel movements, reduce the risk of type 2 diabetes, and help with weight control by making you feel fuller longer.

Your culinary experiences with oats may be limited to the breakfast table, but this hearty grain can go beyond the cereal bowl. Make a side dish with steel-cut oats, vegetables, and herbs, use oats in homemade nutrition bars or pancakes, or mix them into a nut loaf or veggie burgers. You can also substitute oat flour (create your own by chopping rolled oats in a blender or food processor) for some of the wheat flour in your favorite recipes.

Quinoa

Quinoa has quickly climbed the ranks from the unrecognizable and hard-to-pronounce grain (KEEN-wah) to the top tier among mainstream grains in the supermarket. Quinoa dates back thousands of years, when it served as a staple and sacred food for the Incans in Peru and Bolivia.

This ancient grain contains a cache of important nutrients: One half-cup of cooked quinoa contains 4 grams of protein (it is one of the few plant foods that provides significant amounts of all nine essential amino acids in one serving), 5 grams of fiber, and several B vitamins, iron, magnesium, zinc, and copper.

While quinoa is relatively new to the world of nutrition research, some studies document its potential antioxidant and anti-inflammatory benefits and its role in managing diabetes, helping control blood pressure, and aiding with weight control by keeping you feeling fuller longer. What's more, quinoa is a gluten-free grain, making it a nutrient-dense alternative for people who must avoid gluten because of celiac disease or gluten sensitivity.

Quinoa is available in shades of ivory, red, and black (or a rainbow combination of these), and it's one of the quickest-cooking whole grains: It cooks up in just 15 minutes. Simmer quinoa in water or broth, and stir it into casseroles and stews or use it as a base for a healthy grain salad to take to potlucks and picnics. Combine cooked quinoa with herbs, onions, and nuts for a savory filling to stuff into bell peppers, acorn squash, or summer squash "boats." Make a nutritious "bowl" lunch by layering cooked quinoa with an assortment of fresh veggies, canned beans or lentils, and a flavorful vinaigrette. Or mix quinoa with chopped spinach, seasonings, and ground nuts or flaxseed to make veggie patties. Quinoa flour also can be used as a gluten-free alternative to wheat flour in baking.

Barley

Barley is one of the first cultivated grains recorded in human history, dating back more than 10,000 years ago to Southwest Asia. It's also a sustainable grain, with a low carbon footprint that's becoming increasingly valuable in our changing climate.

Barley kernels are protected by a tight-fitting, inedible hull. Hulled barley has had the hull removed in a process that causes minimal bran loss, so this form is always a whole grain. Hulless barley is a different variety of barley that grows without a tight hull and is also considered a whole grain. Pearled barley is put through a process called "pearling," which polishes the kernels and removes the hull and the bran layer. Pearled barley is not a whole grain, although it still has a fairly high fiber content.

Barley flakes are similar in appearance to rolled oats; they're made by steaming the barley kernels and then rolling and drying them. Barley flakes are considered a whole grain if they are made from hulled or hulless barley, but not when made from pearled barley.

Hulled barley provides a large dose of fiber—8 grams per serving (about one-half cup cooked), which is higher than most other whole grains. Barley is also one of the two best sources (along with oats) of beta glucan, a type of dietary fiber linked with health benefits, such as promoting gut health, lowering total cholesterol levels, and improving glucose levels. In addition, barley provides a significant amount of protein (6 grams) per serving, as well as thiamin, niacin, iron, magnesium, and selenium.

Barley is probably best known for its use in traditional vegetable or beef soups, but you can also use it instead of rice in dishes like pilafs, stir-fries, curries, and casseroles. Or create a breakfast power bowl by topping cooked barley with cinnamon, raisins, and almonds.

Millet

Millet may be a lesser-known grain to Americans, but it is mentioned in records from ancient Greece and Rome and medieval Europe, as well as in the Old Testament. Each one-half cup of cooked millet serving provides 3 grams of protein and 8 grams of fiber, as well as several vitamins, minerals, and phytochemicals known for their antioxidant and anti-inflammatory properties. While there is limited research documenting specific health benefits of consuming millet, research suggests that it can help with blood glucose and cholesterol control.

Millet can be eaten as a simple breakfast porridge, as is common in Africa, or in *roti*, a traditional Indian bread made with ground millet. Millet can be steamed and served in place of rice to accompany stir-fries or curries, stirred into grain and vegetable salads, used in veggie "meatballs," and added to breads and baked goods. Millet is gluten-free, so it's a good choice for anyone who has celiac disease or gluten sensitivity.

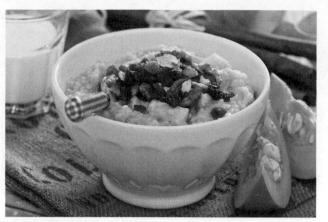

© Fahrwasser | Dreamstime

Try millet porridge topped with nuts and raisins as an alternative to oatmeal.

Teff

Teff holds claim to being the smallest grain in the world, but it's a powerful source of nutrition. Cultivated in Ethiopia since prehistoric times, teff has been the principal source of nutrition for an estimated two-thirds of Ethiopians for centuries; it's the main ingredient in the Ethiopian fermented flatbread called *injera*. It's also a popular staple in other parts of Africa because of its nutrient-dense profile and easy cultivation.

This grain is particularly rich in calcium compared to other grains, providing 10 percent of the recommended daily intake in a one-half cup cooked serving. Teff is also a source of vitamin B_6, zinc, protein (7 grams), and fiber (4 grams), and it's high in resistant starch, a type of fiber that may help with blood glucose management, weight control, and digestive health.

Cook this mild-flavored, dark-colored grain and serve it for breakfast, topped with fresh or dried fruit and nuts or seeds. Use teff as the main ingredient in side dishes, stuffing, and grain salads. You might also try teff flour as a gluten-free alternative in recipes for breads, pancakes, and homemade nutrition bars.

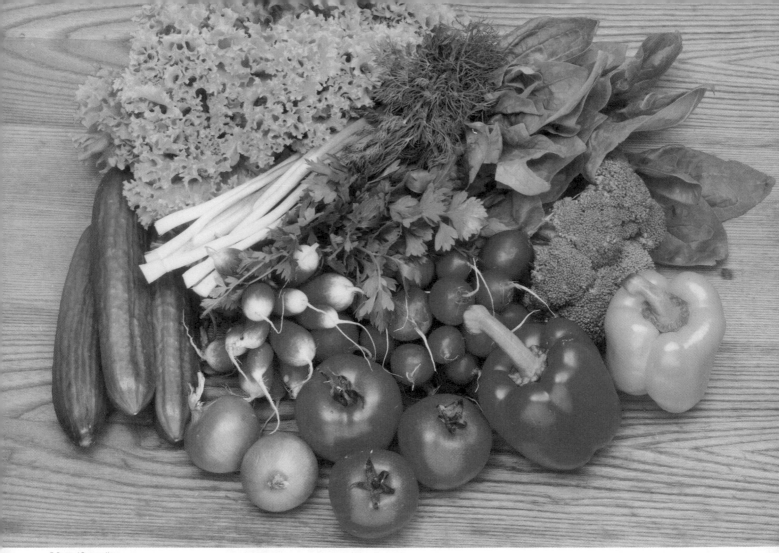

Include a variety of brightly colored vegetables in your daily eating plan to give your body a rich supply of beneficial nutrients.

4 Vegetables

No report on the benefits of superfoods would be complete without a comprehensive section on vegetables, and for good reason. Vegetables are the epitome of "superfoods" due to their superstar nutrient status. Including plenty of these garden-grown wonders in your dietary pattern is tied to a reduced risk of a lengthy list of chronic diseases and conditions. In short, eating vegetables is simply good for you.

Diets plentiful in vegetables are linked with lower risks of cardiovascular disease, type 2 diabetes, several types of cancer, osteoporosis, and obesity. Your brain appears to function better with vegetables, too—research has shown associations between higher vegetable intake and lower incidences of cognitive decline and depression. And eating plenty of vegetables—and fruits—may help you live longer: Researchers who analyzed dietary data from studies involving more than 2 million adults worldwide found that consuming five daily servings of fruits and vegetables was associated with the lowest risk of death.

Vegetables are a "must have" food group in all of the recommended eating patterns recommended in the 2020-2025 *Dietary Guidelines for Americans*. Organizations such as the U.S. Department of Agriculture (USDA) recommend a vegetable intake of about two to three cups each day, varying somewhat based on gender and age. Unfortunately, only about one in 10 Americans meets these recommendations, according to a report issued by the Centers for Disease

Control and Prevention (see "Vegetable, Fruit Consumption Is Very Low Among U.S. Adults").

But choosing vegetables goes beyond quantity: For the best nutrition, select a wide range of colors from the rainbow of vegetable options. Not only will your vegetables be beautiful to look at—think of the gorgeous reds, purples, greens, oranges, and yellows—but they're also loaded with phytonutrients that have been linked with health benefits. For example, blue and purple vegetables contain anthocyanins, red vegetables contain lycopene, and yellow and orange vegetables provide carotenoids.

It's easy to get into a rut and eat the same vegetables week in and week out. To expand your selections, visit a farmers market, where you'll likely find far more than your typical varieties of vegetables. Examples include mint-green fennel and Romanesco cauliflower, purple Brussels sprouts and carrots, and heirloom tomatoes in hues of mustard yellow, forest green, and dusky purple. Global cuisine markets are another way to boost your vegetable IQ with dozens of different greens, squashes, beans, and mushrooms. Even mainstream grocery stores have broadened their vegetable offerings.

Or try a DIY and grow some colorful vegetables in your backyard or in a container garden on your porch or patio (no space is too small!). You may find tomatoes, green beans, squash, broccoli, herbs, and leafy greens even tastier when you've planted, cared for, and harvested them yourself, and they'll have just-picked freshness—not to mention benefiting the environment and your wallet by cutting the number of miles your food travels and the number of dollars you spend.

A simple way to boost your vegetable intake is to include them in almost every meal and snack. Add onions, tomatoes, spinach, or mushrooms, to your breakfast scramble; snack on celery, carrots, and bell peppers with hummus or tahini; use Romaine or Bibb lettuce leaves to wrap up your sandwich filling or veggie burger; and start your evening meal with a vegetable salad or soup—or both. Prepare vegetables with healthy cooking methods, such as roasting, steaming, grilling, or sautéing, and skip cream-based and cheesy sauces. Accentuate vegetables' natural flavors by dressing them with a light drizzle of olive oil, a twist of lemon, and/or a sprinkle of fresh herbs.

Indeed, *all* vegetables are good sources of nutrients, including these common varieties:

- Artichokes
- Asparagus
- Avocado
- Beets
- Broccoli
- Brussels sprouts
- Cabbage
- Carrots
- Cauliflower
- Celery
- Chard
- Corn
- Cucumber
- Eggplant
- Green beans
- Green peas
- Kale
- Leeks
- Lettuce
- Mushrooms
- Okra
- Onions
- Parsnips
- Peppers
- Potatoes
- Radishes
- Spinach
- Squash
- Sweet potatoes
- Tomatoes
- Turnips

Top Picks

You'll gain health benefits from eating any type of vegetable, but here are some standouts that top the superfoods list.

Avocados

Avocados have a rich, creamy, almost buttery texture, and they're high in monounsaturated fat, one of the healthy fats linked with protective effects on the heart and vascular system.

One ounce of avocado (about one-fifth of a medium avocado) contains a modest 45 calories and many health-protective nutrients, such as vitamins C, E, and K, folate, phytosterols, and phytochemicals

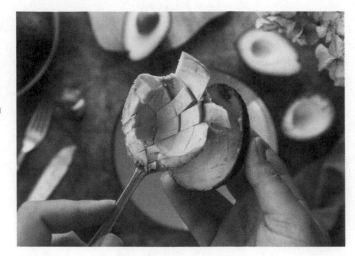

Here's a quick and easy way to make avocado cubes: Score the avocado with a knife in a crisscross pattern before scooping out the flesh.

© Erhaninga85 | Dreamstime

such as beta-carotene and lutein. Studies show that including avocados in your diet can help with weight control, thanks to a generous dose of fiber and healthy fat, which can help increase satiety. Additionally, intake of avocados may be associated with cardioprotective benefits (see "Avocados Linked to Lower Incidence of Heart and Vascular Disease"). Another bonus is that, when you add avocados to a salad or a meal, the fat they provide helps your body better absorb the fat-soluble vitamins A, D, E, and K.

It's easy to incorporate avocados into your dietary pattern. Make avocado toast for breakfast or a snack: Just mash ripe avocados to create an avocado "butter" and spread it on whole-grain toast. Add more nutrients by topping it with sliced tomatoes, fresh basil or other herbs, or a sprinkle of chopped nuts or seeds. On sandwiches or bagels, replace mayonnaise or cream cheese with avocado "butter." Include avocado slices or chunks in salads, omelets, burritos, and tacos. Adding avocados to smoothies will give them a creaminess as well as a nutrient boost. And, of course, there's the ever-popular guacamole dip.

Asparagus

When those tender spears of asparagus first pop out of the soil to greet the spring sunshine, it's a harbinger of good taste and health. Asparagus contains more folate, a B vitamin, per serving than any other vegetable, which is especially important for women who are pregnant, since folate can help prevent birth defects in the fetus, as well as reduce the risk of premature birth. Folate is also needed for the formation of red blood cells.

Asparagus is a source of fiber, other B vitamins, potassium, selenium, manganese, zinc, and iron—all for just 40 calories per one-cup serving. This green vegetable contains powerful plant compounds: rutin, which helps strengthen capillary walls; glutathione, the "master" antioxidant that supports immune system function and aids in removing toxins from your body; the fiber inulin, which is known for feeding healthy gut bacteria; and saponins, which have been linked to blood glucose and cholesterol control. Some studies suggest that asparagus may have anticancer properties and heart-health benefits.

Easy ways to prepare asparagus, available in green, purple, and white varieties, include steaming, roasting, and grilling; finish it with a drizzle of extra-virgin olive oil, a sprinkle of freshly ground pepper, and a squeeze of lemon juice. Asparagus also can be

NEW FINDING

Avocados Linked to Lower Incidence of Heart and Vascular Disease

Replacing other fat-containing foods with avocado may help reduce risk for cardiovascular disease, researchers say. The study included data from 68,786 women from the Nurses' Health Study and 41,701 men from the Health Professionals Follow-up Study who were free from cancer, coronary heart disease, and stroke at study baseline. Dietary data were collected utilizing food frequency questionnaires at baseline and then every four years for up to 30 years of follow-up. Analyses showed that the study participants who consumed two or more servings of avocados per week had 16 percent lower risk of cardiovascular disease and 21 percent lower risk of coronary heart disease than participants who didn't consume avocados. In this study, one serving of avocado was one-half cup. Additionally, the researchers noted that replacing even half a serving of margarine, butter, egg, yogurt, cheese, or processed meat with half a serving of avocado was linked with a 16 to 22 percent lower risk of cardiovascular disease.

Journal of the American Heart Association, March 30, 2022

diced into risottos, stir-fries, and pasta dishes, or puréed into a creamy soup. For the best flavor and texture, cook this delicate vegetable only until it is bright green and crisp-tender.

Leafy Green Vegetables

Leafy green vegetables are included in virtually every healthy eating pattern recommended by nutrition and health experts. From spinach and kale to little gem lettuce and rainbow chard, leafy green vegetables are very low in calories: A one-cup serving of spinach provides just seven calories, a cup of shredded Romaine provides eight calories, and a cup of kale has about 30 calories.

Low calories do not equate with low nutrient content, however: Leafy greens provide at least 19 essential nutrients, including vitamins C and K, potassium, magnesium, iron, and folate. In addition, many contain calcium that is needed for bone health. Leafy green vegetables are rich in disease-fighting phytochemicals, such as beta-carotene, betalains, chlorophyll, kaempferol, lutein, quercetin, and zeaxanthin. Some leafy green vegetables, such as kale, collard and turnip greens, and arugula, are members of the cruciferous family of vegetables.

Eating more leafy green vegetables has been linked with multiple health benefits, including protection against cancer, osteoporosis, memory decline, and age-related eye disease. Leafy green vegetables are also a source of vitamin K, which may have cardioprotective benefits (see "Vitamin K May Help Protect Against Atherosclerotic CVD"). The USDA MyPlate guide suggests including one-and-a-half to two cups of green vegetables in your diet each week.

The heartier varieties of leafy greens, such as kale, spinach, and mustard greens, can be quickly sautéed with garlic, stirred into pasta dishes and soups, or blended into pesto. Try filling collard and Romaine leaves with tuna or chicken salad, grilled tofu, or refried beans and brown rice.

One simple way to guarantee you're getting valuable nutrients is to eat a green salad most days of the week. Make salads more nutritious by adding other fresh vegetables or fruit, as well as nuts or seeds, and dress them with tasty vinaigrettes made with your favorite olive oil and vinegar. But skip the cheese, bacon, croutons, and creamy dressings that will weigh the salad down with extra calories and saturated fat.

Broccoli

Broccoli perfectly embodies the superpowers of the cruciferous vegetable family, which also includes cabbage, Brussels sprouts, cauliflower, kale, and collard greens. One cup of raw broccoli provides more than 100 percent of the recommended daily amounts of vitamins C and K, as well as vitamin A, folate, and fiber. In addition, broccoli and other cruciferous vegetables contain phytochemicals called glucosinolates, which have cancer-fighting potential.

In addition to reducing inflammation and oxidative stress, including broccoli in your diet may help promote healthy digestion, prevent bone density loss, and contribute to a healthy cardiovascular system.

Broccoli is very versatile; enjoy the florets dipped in hummus or other bean-based dips, thinly chop or grate the stalks for use in salads and slaws, roast it with a touch of olive oil and balsamic vinegar for a side dish, or sauté it with bell peppers, onions, and carrots in a stir-fry. Along with broccoli, include a variety of other cruciferous vegetables in your weekly meal plan: Toss cauliflower florets with hot sauce to make a "Buffalo-style" dish, caramelize Brussels sprouts by roasting them in the oven, and mix chopped kale into green salads and soups.

NEW FINDING

Vitamin K May Help Protect Against Atherosclerotic CVD

Consuming foods that contain vitamin K (vitamin K_1, from green leafy vegetables and vegetable oils, and vitamin K_2, from fermented foods, eggs, cheese, and chicken) may contribute to a reduced risk of atherosclerosis (plaque buildup in the arteries) and resulting cardiovascular disease (CVD) and related events, including heart disease and peripheral artery disease, myocardial infarction (heart attack), and stroke. Dietary and medical data were collected from more than 53,000 participants and tracked over a 21-year period in the Danish Diet, Cancer, and Health study. Participants with the highest intake of vitamin K_1 had a 21 percent lower risk of hospitalization due to CVD compared to those with the lowest intake. Similarly, risk for hospitalization due to CVD was 14 percent lower for participants with the highest intake of vitamin K_2 compared to those in the lowest intake groups.

Journal of the American Heart Association, Aug. 7, 2021

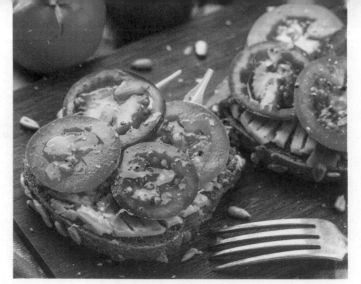

Tomatoes

Tomatoes are the No. 1 non-starchy vegetable consumed in the United States, second in popularity only to potatoes. There are more than 10,000 varieties of tomatoes, including many colorful heirloom varieties, such as Arkansas Traveler, Black Russian, Mr. Stripey, and White Beauty, that have been passed down through generations. With such diverse global variety and culinary uses, tomatoes are an obvious staple in the American kitchen.

Tomatoes are rich in powerful nutrients, including vitamins A, B_6, C, and K, potassium, and manganese. In addition, red tomatoes are the richest source of the phytochemical lycopene in the U.S. diet. Lycopene—the plant compound that lends tomatoes their distinctive, red-orange hue—has attracted the attention of nutrition scientists for its powerful antioxidant and anti-inflammatory actions. In particular, eating a few servings a week of tomatoes may help protect against prostate cancer and possibly breast cancer, as well as heart disease and stroke, UV-related skin damage, osteoporosis, and lung disease. Research also suggests that low-calorie, high-fiber tomatoes may aid in weight loss.

In the case of tomatoes, fresh is not always best: When tomatoes are cooked, the lycopene has a higher bioavailability, meaning that it is more easily absorbed and used by your body. (Tomato products are cooked as part of the preserving process.) Keep your pantry stocked with plenty of low-sodium or no-salt-added canned and jarred tomato varieties—sauce, paste, stewed, crushed, puréed, diced—as well as tomato-based soups and salsas. In addition, lycopene is more absorbable in the presence of fat, so include olive oil in dishes you make with tomatoes.

Including tomatoes and tomato products in your diet is easy—just stir tomato sauce or canned tomatoes into soups, stews, pasta and rice dishes, and casseroles. Put sliced tomatoes on sandwiches or veggie burgers; sprinkle diced tomatoes on tacos, omelets, or bean dip; stir them into homemade guacamole, hummus, or curries; and keep cherry or grape tomatoes on hand to enjoy as a fresh snack or to toss into salads.

Beets

Thanks to a recently renewed culinary appreciation, beets have gone from boring cellar food to fabulous feature on restaurant menus. The vibrant, deep red color of beets comes from the phytonutrient betacyanin, which has been found to have anticancer effects. In addition, beets are a good source of dietary fiber, folate, potassium, magnesium, manganese, and vitamin C—all for only 74 calories per cup cooked. Beets also contain betaine, an amino acid shown to lower inflammation in the body.

Research shows that beets may help fight heart disease by reducing LDL ("bad") cholesterol and increasing HDL ("good") cholesterol levels, as well as reducing blood pressure levels.

Try roasting beets (with onions and/or carrots if you desire) in the oven and serving them with a drizzle of balsamic vinegar and extra-virgin olive oil and a sprinkle of salt-free seasoning. Or make a vegetarian version of the classic Russian dish *borscht* (beet soup). Raw beets have a crunchy, sweet flavor; after peeling, shred or shave them into a green salad or slaw. To broaden your culinary horizons, try heirloom beets that come in an array of colors, such as gold, yellow, pink, white, and pink and white striped.

Squash

Squashes are one of the most important food staples in the traditional Native American diet. Summer squashes have softer skins and flesh and must be eaten shortly after harvest. Winter squashes are hardier, with tough outer skins that can preserve them for months if they're stored in a cool, dry location.

Varieties of summer squashes include zucchini, pattypan, crookneck, and tatuma, a Mexican heirloom squash. You'll find even more color and diversity among winter squashes, which include acorn, butternut, Hubbard, banana, spaghetti, turban, and kabocha varieties. Pumpkins also belong to the squash family.

The flesh of squash is packed with slow-digesting carbs, fiber, essential vitamins and minerals, and phytochemicals. The nutrient profile depends on the type of squash. Summer squashes are very low in calories (about 20 per one-cup raw serving) and are generally rich in vitamin C, B vitamins, fiber, magnesium, manganese, and potassium. Phytochemicals in summer squashes include lutein and zeaxanthin, which help protect vision. Winter squashes are a bit higher in carbohydrates and calories, providing about 75 calories in a one-cup cooked serving. Winter squashes are typically rich in vitamins A, B_6, C, and K, as well as fiber, manganese, copper, potassium, and folate.

Phytonutrient compounds common among varieties of winter squashes include alpha-carotene, beta-carotene, lutein, zeaxanthin, and beta-cryptoxanthin. Research suggests that the nutrients in squash provide protection

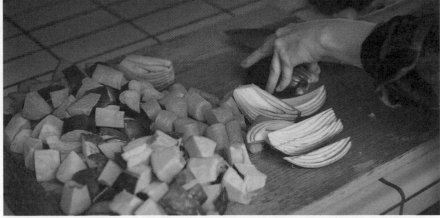

© Yobro10 | Dreamstime

against cancer and cardiovascular disease, and may contribute to healthy blood pressure and blood sugar levels and a longer life.

Serve summer squashes raw as crudités with a yogurt dip, sautéed and added to a breakfast scramble, or grilled on skewers with onions and mushrooms. They can be crafted into "boats" for a special dinner or occasion; cut them in half, scoop out the seeds, fill with seasoned buckwheat, brown rice, or cornbread stuffing, and bake. Winter squashes (including pumpkins) are delicious roasted, puréed in creamy soups, and added to curry dishes. Cutting into a winter squash can be challenging; microwaving the squash or pumpkin for 3 to 5 minutes before cutting will help soften it up.

Carrots

You may think of sweet, crispy carrots for their bright, sunny hue, yet today's standard, orange-colored carrot is a relatively recent creation in the history of carrot cultivation. The first domesticated carrots were purple, yellow, red, and white. Multi-colored "heirloom" carrots are now routine offerings in supermarkets and farmers markets, and they're a great addition to home gardens. Regardless of their color, these root vegetables have much to offer in terms of flavor and health.

Orange carrots are very high in vitamin A. Carrots of all colors also contain notable amounts of fiber, potassium, and vitamins B_6, C, and K. Carrot consumption has been linked to better

For an easy superfoods side dish, cut squash and carrots into cubes, slice onions, toss with olive oil, place on a baking sheet, and bake for 30-40 minutes until vegetables are fork-tender.

cardiovascular health and protection from cancer and eye diseases that can cause vision loss.

In addition, carrots have a variety of phytochemicals linked to their different shades: Orange carrots are highest in beta-carotene, yellow carrots have more lutein, and purple carrots provide anthocyanidins.

Roast carrots alone or with other root vegetables for a caramelization that creates a satisfying mix of sweet and savory flavors. Carrots will add texture and flavor to soups, stews, and stir-fries. Mix shredded raw carrots into slaws and salads, and stir them into your morning oatmeal or porridge. Snack healthy by pairing carrot sticks and other fresh veggies with hummus, bean-based dips, or tahini. You can also add grated carrots to muffin, cake, and bread batters.

Onions

Onions are superfoods that are easily overlooked, since they're used in so many dishes. Yet their nutritional contributions are notable: Every time you make a recipe that includes onions, you are not only getting their trademark pungent aromas and flavors, but also their unique healthful properties, to your meal.

Onions are a member of the *Allium* vegetable family, which also includes garlic, leeks, green onions, chives, and shallots. These foods contain a number of organosulfur compounds that contribute those trademark flavors and odors, as well as antioxidant activity linked with protection against cancer and heart disease. Onions also provide manganese, vitamins B and C, folate, potassium, and the phytochemical quercetin.

There are a variety of onions to explore for different flavors and textures: Choose from white, yellow, red, green, and purple. Many trademark dishes start with sautéed onions, including spicy Indian curries, Italian pasta sauces, and French foods that begin with the flavor base *mirepoix*—a combination of sautéed onions, carrots, and celery.

Add an "invisible" serving of vegetables to your daily diet simply by starting with an onion when making a casserole, soup, or pasta sauce. Fresh onions can brighten up a green or grain salad, sandwich, or bowl of chili, and sautéed onions, which caramelize and sweeten when cooked slowly, can add another layer of flavor to breakfast scrambles and turkey or veggie burgers.

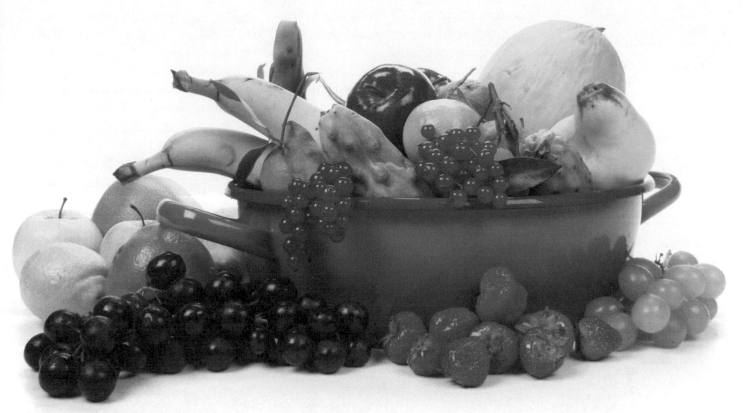

Fruits provide phytonutrients, substances that have been linked with a number of health-protective effects.

5 Fruits

For people working to improve their overall diet and boost their nutrient intake, one of the simplest, easiest, and tastiest ways to make a change is by increasing their fruit intake. With increased accessibility to fruit options from grocery shops, farmers markets, and from "imperfect produce" delivery companies, fruit choices can be plentiful, satisfying, and part of an overall healthy eating pattern.

In addition to being nature's sweet treats, fruits provide a powerful nutritional punch—they are rich in a wide range of health-promoting vitamins, such as vitamin C and folate, and minerals, like potassium and magnesium. Fruits can also help you stay hydrated, since they have a high water content.

Fruits are plentiful sources of phytonutrients—compounds in plants that have been linked to many health benefits as well as disease prevention. Consuming a range of different fruits helps ensure intake of phytonutrients such as carotenoids, which may help support eye health and immune health, and flavonoids, which may be protective against certain types of cancer and cardiovascular disease. Some fruits, especially grapes and grape skin, are sources of resveratrol, a compound associated with the support of cardiovascular health and cognitive function.

Replacing traditional, sugar-sweetened desserts, which are associated with increased risks of obesity, heart disease, diabetes, and other chronic health problems, with fruits allows you to enjoy those sweet, juicy flavors guilt-free. And the fiber in fruits helps decrease the rate at which the natural sugars are broken down, which helps prevent spikes in blood sugar levels.

Choosing fruits as a meal ender (aka "dessert") is an often-recommended tip for people who are working to improve their overall nutrition. Whether the

Goji Berries May Boost "Good" HDL Cholesterol

Results from a 16-week randomized controlled trial of middle-aged and older adults tested the impact of consuming goji berries on vascular outcomes and cardiovascular disease (CVD) risk factors. Study participants were randomly assigned to follow either a healthy dietary pattern (control group) or a healthy dietary pattern plus 15 grams of whole, dried goji berries each day. At the end of the study period, the group that consumed the goji berries had significantly higher HDL ("good") cholesterol than the control group, along with lower predicted long-term CVD risk. Additional studies are needed to learn more about the effects of consuming goji berries on vascular health and CVD risk.

The American Journal of Clinical Nutrition, July 2021

person's goal is to make dietary changes for weight loss or to help stave off the development of chronic disease, the consumption of fruit in place of sugary dessert foods can help reduce one's overall sugar and calorie intake. The dietary fiber present in fruits may also help to increase feelings of fullness, which can have beneficial impacts on future food choices and intake.

Research links fruit consumption of all varieties—fresh, canned, frozen, or dried, with no added sugar—to numerous health benefits, such as lowering the risk of high blood pressure, heart disease, stroke, cancer, eye disease, type 2 diabetes, obesity, diverticulitis, chronic obstructive pulmonary disease (COPD), and neurodegenerative diseases. One study found that diets higher in fruits were linked with better protection of cognitive function. Additionally, analysis of data from the National Health and Nutrition Examination Survey (NHANES), in which dietary recall data from more than 25,000 people was collected, reported a link between dried fruit, nutrient intake, and diet quality. The researchers noted that 7.2 percent of participants who consumed dried fruit had overall higher quality diets and lower body mass indices (BMI), waist circumference, and blood pressure than those who did not. The USDA MyPlate guide suggests that adults consume one-and-a-half to two cups of fruit per day as part of a healthy eating plan, depending on age and gender.

It's important to note that *every* fruit is a superfood. Your goal should be to include a variety of fruits in your diet every day. Commonly available fruits include:

- Apples
- Apricots
- Bananas
- Blackberries
- Blueberries
- Boysenberries
- Cantaloupe
- Cherries
- Cranberries
- Dates
- Figs
- Grapefruit
- Grapes
- Guava
- Honeydew
- Kiwifruit
- Lemons
- Limes
- Mangos
- Nectarines
- Oranges
- Papaya
- Peaches
- Pears
- Persimmons
- Pineapple
- Plums
- Pomegranates
- Raspberries
- Star fruit
- Strawberries
- Watermelon

The Sweetest Selections

The fruits in this section have been linked with particular health benefits in recent scientific studies.

Berries

Berries are the crown jewels of the fruit kingdom. There's much to love about these juicy gems that are one of the most prized fruits around the world. Exotic varieties, such as acai and goji berries, receive a lot of attention for their associated health benefits (see "Goji Berries May Boost 'Good' HDL Cholesterol"). Blueberries, blackberries, strawberries, raspberries, lingonberries, and cranberries are also nutritious and grow closer to home in North America. These brightly colored fruits offer delectable flavors and particularly potent health benefits.

In general, berries are high in fiber, potassium, and vitamin C. But of perhaps greater significance, berries are particularly potent in phytochemicals, plant compounds that are associated with better health. Those most studied in berries include anthocyanins and flavonols, which have antioxidant activity; by neutralizing potentially damaging free radicals in the body, they may help prevent some chronic diseases. Many of these compounds also have strong anti-inflammatory effects.

Berries, especially blueberries and strawberries, are some of the most widely researched fruits. Hundreds of studies have linked berries with lower risks of cancer, cardiovascular disease, diabetes, and age-related mental decline. In addition, they have specific benefits, such as blueberries' protective effects on brain health and the cardiovascular system and cranberries' role in helping to prevent urinary tract infections. Recent research also suggests that cranberries may have cardioprotective benefits, especially in men (see "Cranberries May Help Increase Men's Cardiovascular Function"). Another recent study found that raspberries may help reduce the need for insulin in people with prediabetes or insulin resistance.

Make the most of these health-promoting properties by including a serving of colorful berries on your menu at least a few times per week. Color indicates phytochemical content, so the deeper the color, the better. Enjoy them fresh as a snack, mix them into overnight oats, layer them with plain yogurt and granola to create a parfait, and add to green salads or fresh fruit salads. Berries also boost nutrition in smoothies, baked treats, pancakes, and waffles. Reduce your sugar intake by blending or mashing berries to make a natural fruit spread. Since berry season is short in many locations, keep unsweetened frozen or dried berries on hand for a convenient source of powerful phytochemicals.

Citrus

Add a little sunshine and some big health rewards to your day compliments of citrus fruits, such as oranges, grapefruit, tangerines, lemons, and limes, which offer a wealth of nutrients. An array of citrus varieties is available to discover, including Kaffir limes, red-fleshed blood oranges, kumquats, and Pixie tangerines.

The health benefits of citrus fruits have been known for centuries. They are famously rich in the powerful antioxidant vitamin C—a medium orange provides 130 percent of the recommended daily amount.

Previous research has shown that eating vitamin C-rich foods, such as citrus fruit, is linked with the prevention of age-related muscle loss. Researchers analyzed data from the food diaries of more than 13,000 people between 42 and 82 years old, as well as their blood levels of vitamin C, and found that those with the highest amounts of vitamin C in their diet or blood had the greatest skeletal muscle mass, compared to those with the lowest amounts of vitamin C. But citrus fruits' nutrition package goes far beyond vitamin C, including several B vitamins, potassium, calcium, phosphorus, magnesium, copper, and fiber.

In addition, citrus fruit contains more than 170 different types of phytochemicals, such as limonoids, flavonoids, and carotenoids, which vary depending on the type and color of the fruit. Benefits linked to citrus fruits include protection against heart disease, stroke, arthritis, asthma, cognitive decline, and diabetes. One study found that eating an orange a day may significantly reduce the risk of age-related macular degeneration.

Nothing beats the cheerful, bright flavors of citrus fruits and juices when it comes to creating tangy vinaigrettes, marinades, and salsas. If you find plain water boring, adding a few citrus squeezes or slices can make it more appealing. And citrus can even help you reduce your sodium intake: By adding lemon or lime juice and/or zest, you can cut back on the added salt in recipes while retaining good flavor. And lemon juice can brighten the taste and the look of your dishes by preventing the oxidation that turns some fruits brown; squeeze a lemon over sliced avocados, bananas, or apples and toss to coat to keep your fruit looking fresh.

Apples

Apples may be an American staple in dishes like apple pie, but their fame is shared globally. More than 7,500 varieties of this white-fleshed favorite are

NEW FINDING

Cranberries May Help Improve Men's Cardiovascular Function

Cranberries and cranberry juice have been identified as having potential cardiovascular health benefits. A double-blind, randomized controlled trial was completed in 45 healthy men who were randomly assigned to one-month daily consumption of either cranberry (9 grams of powder solubilized in water, equivalent to 100 grams of fresh cranberries containing 525 milligrams of polyphenols) or control (9 grams of a powder containing no polyphenols). Researchers found that regular consumption of cranberry powder was associated with improvements in endothelial function. (The endothelium is a thin layer of cells that lines blood vessels.) Endothelial cells release substances that affect blood vessels' contraction and expansion, as well as blood clotting—functions that impact the risk of developing cardiovascular disease.

Food and Function, March 2022

available, from subtly sweet Red and Golden Delicious to the crisp bite of Braeburn and Fuji to the tart Pippin and Granny Smith (a favorite for cooking). And apples (and other fleshy fruit with seeds, such as pears) can be enjoyed year-round due to a technique called controlled atmosphere storage—which means temperature, oxygen, carbon dioxide, and humidity levels are controlled to lengthen their lifespan.

Although they're high in flavor, nutrients, and chewing satisfaction, apples have a moderate calorie count. One medium apple has 95 calories, and it is high in vitamin C and fiber, including a type of soluble fiber called pectin, which has been shown to lower blood cholesterol and protect against heart disease. In fact, research links apples to numerous health benefits, including weight control, digestive and immune health, cancer prevention, and cardiovascular health.

Apples also contain a phytonutrient called quercetin, which has been linked to slowing down the digestion of carbohydrates, thus improving blood glucose control. The phytonutrient levels in apples vary depending on the variety and color of the apple; for example, red apples contain anthocyanins. Eat the skin to gain the most fiber and phytonutrient content.

You know that apples are famously delicious in baked desserts, including cobblers, tarts, and crostatas, but their sweet-tart flavors also suit savory dishes, such as chicken salad, crunchy slaws, and crisp, green salads. In addition, apples are wonderful paired with yogurt dips, nut and seed butters, and single-serving, low-fat cheeses. While whole apples are the perfect grab-and-go snack, a bumper crop can be cooked down into a delicious sugar-free applesauce or apple butter. Also include apple's close relative, the pear, which is similar in nutritional quality and rich in fiber.

Stone Fruits

Peaches are one of summer's finest gifts, ripe and juicy straight from the tree, or starring in a just-baked crisp or a cool fruit salad. Along with other summer favorites, such as cherries, plums, nectarines, and apricots, peaches are a stone fruit, known for their single large seed, or "stone," at the fruit's center.

There are thousands of varieties of fruits within the category of stone fruits, such as Rainier cherries, Dixie Red peaches, Italian plums, Arctic Rose nectarines, and Autumn Royal apricots, as well as delicious hybrids, such as pluots (plum-apricot) and apriums (apricot-plum). More common varieties may be available in your supermarket during the season, but you'll find more interesting types at your local farmers markets, or even at your local nursery for planting at home.

The nutritional profiles of stone fruits vary depending on the type and variety of fruit, though they are all generally rich in soluble fiber, slow-digesting carbohydrates, vitamin C, potassium, and phytochemicals, at a calorie bargain (about 60 calories per one-half cup serving). Beyond that, each stone fruit brings a little something special. Peaches, nectarines, and apricots are rich in vitamin A, as well as the phytochemicals linked with their colors—carotenoids, anthocyanins, quercetins, and catechins that act as anti-inflammatory and antioxidant agents. Plums are high in vitamin K and the unique phytochemicals neochlorogenic acid and chlorogenic acid, which are powerful antioxidants. Cherries are rich in anthocyanins, which provide their deep-red color.

The evidence-based health benefits of stone fruits are many; they are associated with lower risks of diabetes, metabolic syndrome, and cardiovascular disease. The stone fruits that contain beta-carotene, such as peaches, nectarines, and apricots, are also linked to a lower risk of eye disease. Anthocyanins in cherries have been found to reduce arthritis symptoms, muscle pain, and the incidence of upper respiratory symptoms after exercise, as well as improve parameters of cardiovascular health.

Start your day off with stone fruits by adding them to your morning cereal bowl or low-fat yogurt parfait. Eat them on their own as a healthy snack, or make a relish or salsa to pair with poultry or seafood. Of course, these succulent fruits shine in fruit-based desserts, such as tarts, bars, pies, and cobblers. During summer cookouts, place skewered peach, plum, nectarine, or apricot halves on the grill for a juicy, simple dessert. To enjoy their taste year-round, freeze or dry them, or turn stone fruits into homemade preserves, fruit butters, or fruit leather.

Bananas

Bananas are the perfectly packaged food, all zipped in yellow and sized to stash in a purse or backpack for a satisfying, nutritious go-to snack. It's not surprising that bananas are among the most popular fruits in the U.S.

Bananas originated in Malaysia some 4,000 years ago, but they are now grown primarily in the tropical and subtropical regions of Central and South America. They are unique because they may be picked green from the tree and then allowed to ripen for several days without requiring refrigeration, which makes them easy to transport around the globe.

In every medium banana, you'll get a generous supply of vitamins B_6 and C, potassium, manganese, fiber, and copper. In addition, bananas contain plant sterols linked with heart health, as well as special types of fibers—soluble pectin and fructooligosaccharides, which foster the growth of friendly bacteria in the gut, thus boosting immune function and digestive health. Bananas contain resistant starch, which promotes gut health

by acting as a prebiotic and may help manage diabetes and keep you feeling full longer.

Studies have found that bananas may be an ideal food for athletes, since they are a source of sustained energy and their mineral content aids in preventing muscle cramps. Slice a banana over toast spread with nut butter, whole-grain breakfast flakes, or plain yogurt. Add a banana to a smoothie to give it a thicker, creamier texture. Mashed, very ripe bananas can take the place of added sugars in baked goods and desserts, such as breads, muffins, and cookies. To avoid food waste, peel ripe bananas and store them in the freezer before they spoil.

Mangos

There's nothing like the aromatic, sweet bite of mango to bring to mind a tropical paradise. These golden-fleshed fruits wrapped in varying hues of green, red, and yellow grow in tropical climates. There are more than 1,000 mango varieties, but the ones you see in your supermarket typically hail from Mexico, Ecuador, Peru, Brazil, Guatemala, and Haiti.

Look past mango's vibrant color and sweet flavor to its nutrient profile, and you'll find a fruit that's very high in vitamin C that also provides fiber, vitamins A and B_6, folate, and copper. In addition, mangos are packed with phytochemicals, including ellagic acid, gallotannin, and the unique compound mangiferin. Research has linked mango intake to improved glucose control, better bone health, and possible cancer-protective effects.

Make the most of the tropical taste of mangos by enjoying them with granola or yogurt and in a fruit salad. (Mango skin contains urushiol, the same substance as in poison ivy, so be sure to remove all of the skin; you also may want to rinse the mango before eating it.) Try mango puréed in smoothies and

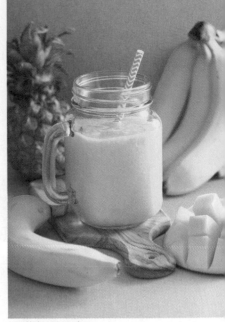

© Duskbabe | Dreamstime

For a double dose of superfoods fruits, combine bananas and mangos in a sunny smoothie that's high in fiber and antioxidants.

fruit sorbets or frozen into healthy pops for hot summer days. Serve a mango salsa or relish as an accompaniment for grilled fish or as an appetizer served with whole-grain crackers.

Choose mangos that are mostly yellow and/or red in color; green mangos generally are not ripe. Mangos should give slightly when you gently squeeze them, but they should not be mushy. You can find fresh mangos almost year-round, and you can usually find mangos in the freezer section of most grocery stores.

Melons

Nothing beats biting into a sweet, juicy slice of watermelon on a hot summer day. But beyond those classic outdoor picnics and parties, melons are also great for snacking, recipes, and helping satisfy a sweet tooth. Some of the most popular varieties include watermelon (which also come in yellow varieties), honeydew, and cantaloupe, yet a much broader variety of melons are available in farmers markets, such as Galia, Canary, Crenshaw, and Horned melons. These varieties offer a wide diversity of color and flavor.

That juicy flesh is a reminder that eating melons can help keep you hydrated due to their high fluid content—they contain up to 90 percent water. Melons are typically low in calories (about 60 calories per cup) and rich in vitamins A and C and potassium, in addition to a variety of phytochemicals. For example, orange-fleshed melons are rich in beta-carotene, and red watermelon contains heart-healthy lycopene and the amino acid citruline, which is linked with heart health. These phytochemicals help furnish melons with their antioxidant and anti-inflammatory actions, which help protect health in numerous ways.

Melons are best enjoyed fresh and simple: Split open a melon, scoop out the seeds, slice into wedges or bite-sized chunks, and enjoy. Melons pair particularly well with the tangy acidity of lime and the pop of fresh mint or ginger. Purée melons into frozen sorbets and smoothies, or dice them and combine with onions, lime juice, and cilantro to make salsa that is an excellent accompaniment for grilled poultry or fish.

Pomegranates

The pomegranate is a symbol of abundant life and vitality in many cultures and is mentioned in ancient texts around the world. Pomegranates are notable for their inclusion in healthy food traditions and celebrations throughout history, such as religious holidays and weddings, as well as folk medicine for healing all manner of ailments, such as infections and indigestion.

Beneath that leathery outer covering and white, fleshy internal substance called albedo, you'll find the edible gems: ruby-colored arils (seeds surrounded by juice sacs), plump with sweet-tart juice. One serving (one-half cup of arils) provides 72 calories, along with a rich supply of the antioxidant vitamin C, vitamin K, potassium, and fiber.

Pomegranate's phytochemicals, which appear to protect the body against the damaging effects of free radicals, are of particular interest to nutrition researchers. These phytochemicals include punicalagin, anthocyanins, ellagitannins, and resveratrol—the same antioxidant compound found in red wine. Studies suggest that pomegranates may be helpful in protecting against high blood pressure, high cholesterol, high blood sugar, some cancers, and cognitive decline. Pomegranate arils may be enjoyed on their own as a snack, or stirred into a salsa or grain dish, sprinkled over salads, muesli, or hummus, or as a gorgeous garnish for most any sweet or savory dish.

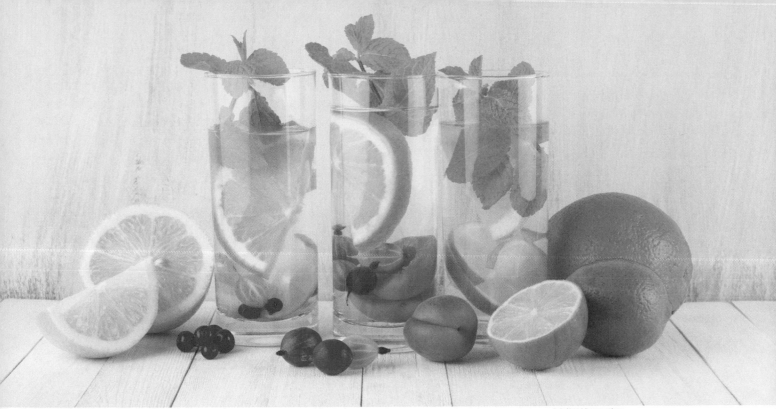

6 Beverages

Beverage choices used to be simpler, in part, because the available options were limited. Now, in an environment of coffee shops, juice bars, and energy-drink-sponsored events, the question of what to drink seems to be a lot more complicated. So many options! How could a person possibly choose between the various "blended-mocha-vanilla-caramel-cinnamon" coffee and tea drinks, the cute and interesting bubble tea varieties, or the energy-boosting promise that comes with a can of the latest caffeinated, carbonated tonic?

Unfortunately, calorie-laden, sugar-sweetened beverages (SSBs, including soft drinks, energy drinks, and fruit drinks) and sweetened teas and coffees contribute few, if any, valuable nutrients to Americans' diets. What they do contribute is plenty of unneeded added sugar; in fact, these SSBs provide more than 40 percent of the U.S. daily intake of added sugars. In recent years, added sugars have gotten more attention from nutrition and health experts, and study after study has linked excess added sugar consumption with a long list of health problems, including increased rates of type 2 diabetes, heart disease, fatty liver disease, depression, obesity, and premature aging.

When consumed, SSBs pump refined sugar into the body, which is rapidly absorbed and causes a spike in blood glucose level. These beverages often come with a high calorie count—150 calories and up per 12-ounce portion. Over time, frequent, regular consumption of SSBs will likely contribute to considerable weight gain.

A study from 2020 reported that calories may not be the only reason SSBs are a leading cause of obesity: They may also affect the hormones that stave off hunger and regulate appetite. When study participants consumed drinks that contained sucrose, a form of added sugar, they produced lower amounts of hormones that suppress hunger than when they consumed drinks containing glucose, a type of sugar found in natural foods like fruits. In addition, drinking a beverage—even if it is high in calories,

Stick to beverages like water, tea, and coffee, and skip the sugary beverages that provide nothing but empty calories.

Coffee Consumption Is Associated with Lower Rates of Mortality

Researchers in Korea have investigated the effects of drinking coffee on mortality (death) rates in a large-scale prospective study. The participants, 173,209 people ages 40 years and older, were enrolled in the study for a median of 9.1 years. Food frequency questionnaires were used to assess coffee consumption. A cup of coffee was defined as 5.1 fluid ounces, and participants were divided into groups according to patterns of consumption: non-consumers, one or fewer cups of coffee per day, one to three cups per day, and more than three cups per day. Participants who drank more than three cups of coffee per day had a lower risk of death from any cause compared to non-consumers, and those who consumed less than or equal to three cups of coffee per day had a reduced risk of death from cardiovascular causes compared to non-consumers.

Journal of the Academy of Nutrition and Dietetics, November 2021

or even fat or fiber—doesn't elicit the same sense of satiety or satisfaction in your brain as it does when you eat solid foods that contain the same amount of calories and nutrients.

Another drawback of including SSBs in your dietary pattern is that you may be missing out on more nutritious alternatives that you might otherwise choose. In addition, sweet drinks are often paired with highly processed foods, including snack foods and fast foods that have few, if any, beneficial nutrients. Making healthier beverage choices may also influence healthier meal and snack selections.

The healthiest beverage choice is good, old-fashioned water, straight from the tap. (Skip the bottled water—you'll save money while reducing your impact on the planet.) You can also enjoy other plant-based, sugar-free choices. In fact, several health benefits have been linked to tea and coffee consumption. Read on to learn what the latest research shows about drinking coffee, tea—and even red wine.

Stay Hydrated

Adequate hydration is an essential ingredient for good health. You need fluids for many physical functions, including maintaining your internal temperature and blood pressure, cushioning joints and organs, facilitating the digestion, absorption, and transport of nutrients, and ridding your body of toxins. To get enough water each day, follow these general guidelines from the National Academy of Sciences:

♦ **Women are advised to consume a total of 2.7 liters** (91 ounces, or the equivalent of about 11 8-ounce glasses) of water from beverages and foods each day.

♦ **Men are advised to consume a total of 3.7 liters** (125 ounces, or the equivalent of about 16 8-ounce glasses) of water from beverages and foods each day.

You can help meet your hydration needs beyond the water glass, though. While about 80 percent of people's water comes from drinking water and beverages, about 20 percent comes from foods. Many foods have a high water content. In fact, most fruits and vegetables, including apples, carrots, grapes, green peas, watermelon, lettuce, pineapple, and spinach, are more than 80 percent water by weight. And many foods that are more than 50 percent water by weight may surprise you—they include cooked pasta and rice, as well as poultry, fish, beef, and eggs.

Coffee

There's never been a better time to be a coffee drinker: Mounting evidence suggests coffee intake is linked with lower rates of mortality (see "Coffee Consumption Is Associated with Lower Rates of Mortality"). Coffee consumption is also related to lower risks of type 2 diabetes and Parkinson's disease, longer life, and better heart health. One review of multiple studies concluded that drinking one or more cups of black, caffeinated coffee a day was associated with a reduced long-term risk of heart failure. In one study, the participants' risk for heart failure over time decreased between 5 percent and 12 percent for each 8-ounce cup of coffee consumed each day. In another study, drinking two or more cups of coffee per day was linked with a 30 percent lower risk of heart failure.

Coffee beans are packed with phytochemicals—over 1,000 active compounds with antioxidant properties have been identified. Research has linked coffee with a list of health-promoting actions, including improved mental and physical performance, liver protection, and cancer-fighting properties. And, while people with heart disease were once advised against drinking coffee, studies have shown that consuming caffeinated beverages does not result in heartbeat abnormalities that can cause health problems for most people.

For some people, consuming too much caffeine—naturally found in coffee and tea—can have detrimental effects; it may aggravate health conditions, including gastroesophageal reflux disease, migraines, and benign fibrocystic breast disease, and it can cause sleep disturbances. However, if you are sensitive to caffeine, you can still gain antioxidant benefits from decaffeinated coffee and tea.

Many of the "gourmet" coffee and tea drinks now available at specialty shops and in bottles or cans on supermarket shelves can be grouped with the sugar-sweetened drinks that were mentioned at the beginning of this chapter. For example, one variety of 16-ounce specialty coffee contains 54 grams of sugar—more than the total amount of added sugar that is recommended daily—along with 10 grams of saturated fat, which is more than a 4-ounce hamburger made with 80-percent lean ground beef.

Tea

Relaxing with a restorative cup of tea has long been one of the world's favorite pastimes; tea has always had a reputation for contributing to the health of the mind, body, and soul. Tea is a beverage that has been used to treat a number of ailments throughout history—and findings from modern research support the position that sipping tea is a healthy habit.

True tea comes from the *Camellia sinensis* plant. The varieties of tea—green, black, oolong, and white—are determined based upon how the leaves are processed.

- **Green tea** is made from mature tea leaves that are steamed, rolled, and dried after picking. Matcha is a powder made from ground green tea leaves.

- **Black tea** is made from mature tea leaves that are oxidized for two to four hours before processing to create an intense color and flavor.
- **Oolong tea** is made from mature tea leaves that are partially oxidized before processing.
- **White tea** is made from the white, fuzzy buds that are picked while young; the buds are not oxidized prior to processing.

One of the key aspects of tea's healthy nutrition profile is its very high levels of phytochemicals in the form of flavonoids—in particular, catechins such as epigallocatechin gallate, found primarily in green tea, and theaflavins and thearubigins, found in black tea. These flavonoids have been the inspiration for hundreds of studies on the health effects of drinking tea. Research suggests that tea consumption is linked with lower risks of heart disease and certain cancers; protection of oral, bone, eye, and immune health; and even modest metabolic benefits.

Herbal teas may not come from the *Camellia sinensis* plant, but they may still be beneficial to your health, and there's no reason not to include them in your diet if you enjoy them. From lavender and chamomile to hibiscus and peppermint, herbal teas are made from infusions of the leaves, roots, bark, seeds, and flowers of a wide variety of plants that possess unique qualities originating from the phytochemical-rich plant itself, including antimicrobial, antiviral, antioxidant, and anticancer properties.

Enjoy tea as a delicious beverage option throughout the day. If you are sensitive to caffeine, you can choose decaffeinated or herbal teas. Serve hot tea with lemon, or make pitchers of iced tea for warm days. Add mint or slices of fresh orange, lime, cucumber, herbs, berries, or even edible flowers to brighten the flavor without added sugar.

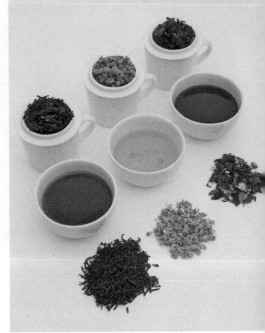

© Duskbabe | Dreamstime

The varying colors and tastes of tea depend on how the tea leaves are processed.

You also can use tea in cooking—concentrated tea infusions and matcha are excellent additions to vinaigrettes, marinades, smoothies, and even baked goods. To reap the most benefits from tea, skip the premade tea drinks and brew your own—the flavonoid contents of freshly brewed teas are much higher than tea drinks in bottles or cans. Making your own tea also means you'll avoid the 4 teaspoons or more of added sugar found in many 8-ounce servings of bottled and canned tea beverages.

Red Wine

If you look forward to sipping a glass of cabernet sauvignon, merlot, or shiraz with dinner, it's reassuring to know that red wine contains compounds that may be good for your health. For thousands of years, red wine has been enjoyed as a celebratory and wholesome part of traditional, healthful diets in much of Europe.

Moderate red wine intake is included in the Mediterranean-style dietary pattern, which is highlighted as one of the three healthy eating patterns recommended by the 2020-2025 *Dietary Guidelines for Americans*. The Mediterranean-style diet has been linked with a host of health benefits, including lower risks of heart disease, diabetes, and neurodegenerative diseases.

Research findings have revealed that moderate consumption of red wine is connected with many specific benefits, including reduced risks of stroke, heart disease, diabetes, multiple sclerosis, Alzheimer's disease, obesity, osteoporosis, and infectious diseases. Overall, enjoying red wine in moderation is associated with lower oxidative stress and healthier aging.

What gives red wine its beneficial qualities? Red wine is rich in phytochemicals that come from grapes—about 200 unique types have been identified, including resveratrol. This phytonutrient has attracted scientists' attention due to its antioxidant, anti-clotting, anti-inflammatory, and anticancer properties. The alcohol in wine also may play a big part in its power; alcohol alone—independent of whether it's found in wine, beer, or spirits—seems to help fight against cardiovascular disease.

The essential factor behind gaining any potential health bonuses in a glass of wine lies in one word: *moderation*. The benefits found in a glass of red wine only occur with moderate consumption—one glass (5 ounces) per day for women, and one to two glasses per day for men. Consuming too much wine—or *any* alcohol, for that matter—can lead to serious health problems, including more than 95,000 annual deaths in the United States related to alcohol consumption. Drinking to excess is associated with neurological disorders, cardiovascular problems, psychological issues, gastrointestinal disorders, and, of course, liver disease. Drinking during pregnancy may cause developmental problems in the fetus. And even moderate alcohol use has been linked with an increased risk of breast and colorectal cancers. In fact, the guidelines stress that it's important to limit alcohol consumption, if you drink at all.

If you already drink wine, do so in moderation, but don't start drinking it just for its potential health benefits. If you have a family history of cancer, you may want to discuss the risks associated with alcohol with your health-care provider.

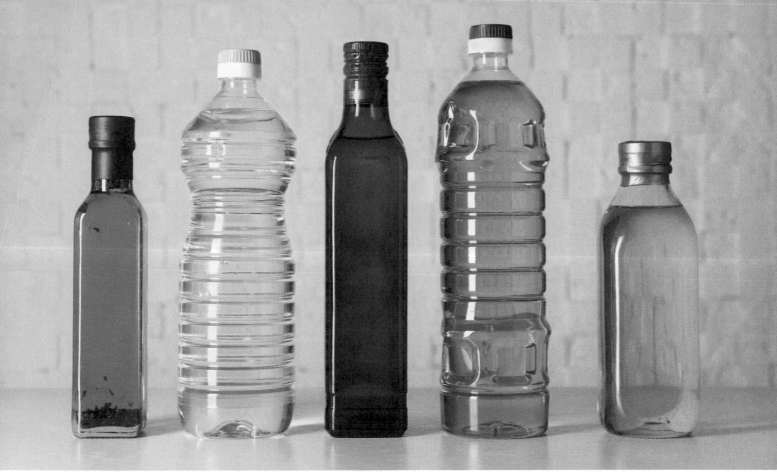

When cooking, use vegetable oils that are high in heart-healthy unsaturated fats.

7 Fats

For many people, the word "fat" used to be synonymous with "bad," since it was believed that rising rates of obesity were due to excessive consumption of high-fat foods. During trips to the grocery store, consumers scrutinized labels looking for the latest fat-free options of their favorite foods, not realizing that these replacements were often similar in total calories and higher in sugar than the original. However, once the low-fat craze had taken hold, researchers began to realize that choosing fat-free or low-fat foods hadn't decreased rates of obesity at all; in fact, rates of obesity continued to rise.

Nowadays, as researchers have learned more about the various types of dietary fats, there is a much better understanding of the relationship between fat intake and health. We now know that dietary fat is essential for overall health. And while health experts don't advise eating as much fat (or as much of anything else) as you want, what's most important to consider may be the types of fats that are consumed rather than the amount that is consumed.

Types of Fats

There are four major dietary fats found in foods: monounsaturated fats (MUFAs), polyunsaturated fats (PUFAs), saturated fats, and trans fats. Intake of MUFAs and PUFAs are considered the healthy fats and the ones to include, whereas saturated fat should be limited, and trans fats (the type that are formed during an industrial process called partial hydrogenation) should be avoided altogether.

MUFAs are present in olive oil, canola oil, peanut oil, safflower oil, sesame oil, avocados, peanut butter, along with many other types of nuts and seeds. PUFAs are often found in plant-based oils such as soybean oil, corn oil, sunflower oil, and in walnuts, sunflower seeds, tofu, soybeans, and fatty fish. MUFAs and PUFAs

FATS	
SOURCE	SATURATED FAT (PER 100 GRAMS)
Palm kernel oil	88.2
Coconut oil	82.5
Palm oil	49.3
Butter	45.6
Lard	39.2
Peanut oil	16.2
Olive oil	15.4
Soybean oil	14.9
Corn oil	13.4
Sunflower oil	8.9
Safflower oil	7.7
Canola oil	6.61

Source: U.S. Department of Agriculture

are considered healthy fats and may help reduce risk of heart disease, especially when used in place of saturated fat.

There are also two major classes of PUFAs, including omega-3 and omega-6 fatty acids—essential fats that the body needs but can't produce for itself. Omega-3 fatty acids are found in pine nuts, walnuts, flaxseed, sunflower seeds, and fatty fish like salmon. Omega-6 fatty acids tend to be in higher percentages in the average diet and are present in safflower oil, sunflower oil, soybean oil, mayonnaise, and salad dressing. Omega-3 and omega-6 are necessary for brain function.

Care should be taken to limit saturated fat intake, due to associated health risks with its consumption. Saturated fat, found in animal foods like beef, poultry, full-fat dairy, eggs, and tropical oils (like coconut, palm, and palm kernel oils) may raise cholesterol levels, negatively impacting cardiovascular health and increasing risk for heart disease. When possible, saturated fat should be replaced with MUFAs or PUFAs.

When industrially produced trans fat was banned from all food products made in the U.S., many food manufacturers replaced it with palm oil. The easiest way to limit foods that contain added saturated fat is to avoid highly processed foods whenever possible—a smart strategy for any healthy eating plan.

Note that industrially produced trans fats are not the same as trans fats that occur naturally at low levels in some animal foods, such as milk, butter, cheese, and meat—these naturally occurring fats have not been linked with harmful health effects.

Healthy Fats in the Kitchen

When you are preparing your daily meals, turn to whole plant foods rich in healthy fats, such as avocados, olives, nuts, seeds, and fatty fish, such as salmon, tuna, and sardines, as your first source of fats in your healthy diet. But which fats should you choose for sautéing vegetables, spreading on your bread, or dressing your salad?

For cooking, your healthiest choices are fats high in PUFAs and MUFAs, such as vegetable oils. Look for salad dressings and plant-based spreads that are low in saturated fat and rich in PUFAs and MUFAs. Replace foods high in saturated fat—butter, shortening, lard, coconut oil—with vegetable oils, with special attention to extra-virgin olive oil. Other good options include canola, soybean, and corn oils, as well as oils extracted from nuts (walnuts, almonds) and seeds (flaxseed, sunflower seeds). In addition, use whole plant foods that contain unsaturated fats, such as avocados, nuts and seeds, and nut and seed butters, more often.

While it's true that your body requires fat to function optimally, keep in mind that fat is a concentrated source of energy. Fat (whether saturated or unsaturated) contains 9 calories per gram, compared to 4 calories per gram for protein and carbohydrates. Just one tablespoon of oil contains 120 calories. If you ladle olive oil into your skillet, top your toast or vegetables with spoonfuls of spread, and douse your vegetable salads with vinaigrette, you'll likely consume far more calories than your body needs, and you may put on extra pounds as a result. You don't need a lot of fat; just a serving (one teaspoon) or two of oils, nuts (about one-quarter cup), seeds (two or three tablespoons), avocados (one-fifth of a medium), or olives (five or six green, black, or kalamata olives) at each meal will get you the healthy fats you need, along with rich, satisfying flavor that will help satisfy your hunger.

Extra-Virgin Olive Oil

Your No. 1 oil in the kitchen should be extra-virgin olive oil (EVOO), the least refined vegetable oil that is commonly available. The olive tree, which dates back at least 6,000 years, has long been a symbol of friendship among nations, and in ancient times, olive branches were awarded to the winners of Olympic games as tokens of victory. For just as many years, the precious oil from olives has been regarded as a health tonic.

We've known for decades that there are evidence-backed health benefits linked with the Mediterranean diet—in which EVOO plays a key role—as well as studies that have revealed strong associations between EVOO and positive health effects.

Benefits of a diet that contains EVOO include a reduced risk of stroke, metabolic syndrome (a constellation of conditions that include unhealthy blood pressure, cholesterol, triglycerides, and dysregulated blood sugar), chronic inflammation, some types of cancer, rheumatoid arthritis, and diseases of the heart and blood vessels (collectively referred to as cardiovascular disease). One study found that people who consumed more EVOO—an average of more than a half a tablespoon per day—had a 14 percent lower risk of cardiovascular disease (CVD) and an 18 percent lower risk of coronary heart disease (CHD) than people who consumed little or no EVOO. In addition, replacing butter, margarine, mayonnaise, or dairy fat with an equivalent amount of olive oil was associated with a 5 to 7 percent lower risk of CVD and CHD. Research has repeatedly demonstrated heart- and cancer-protective effects associated with consuming EVOO each day as part of a traditional Mediterranean diet. Additionally, consumption of EVOO may have beneficial effects on mental health and depression (see "Extra-Virgin Olive Oil May Help Improve Symptoms of Depression").

EVOO is high in MUFAs, and its original bioactive compounds remain largely intact, since it is cold-pressed or expeller-pressed from the olive fruit. (Refined oils have undergone processes that may include heating, chemical solvents, bleaching, and deodorizing; refining creates an oil that has a longer shelf life but has lost most of its phytonutrients.) Olive oil's antioxidant and anti-inflammatory compounds include tyrosol, oleuropein, olecocanthal, and vitamin E.

EVOO is easy to incorporate into your diet. Make it your go-to ingredient in homemade salad dressings and marinades for fish, chicken, and tofu. Use EVOO instead of butter for sautéing, roasting, or grilling vegetables, seafood, tempeh, or turkey burgers. Using EVOO may even boost your intake of nutrients from other healthy foods: Studies have shown that people eat more vegetables with the addition of EVOO, and that many of the nutrients in those vegetables are more easily absorbed when paired with EVOO.

EVOOs offer a variety of flavor profiles—fruity, grassy, buttery, floral, bitter, peppery—depending on the type of olives they're extracted from and the region the olives are grown in, so try different brands to find ones that are most pleasing to your palate. Contrary to popular belief, EVOO *can* be used at higher temperatures, although due to its higher cost and more intense flavor, some people do not use it for cooking. In your supermarket, you'll notice that the EVOO section has expanded steadily over the past few decades, giving you plenty of options. Keep a less expensive EVOO on hand for sautéing and roasting and a higher-quality EVOO on hand for providing distinctive flavor to salads, cooked vegetables, and pasta dishes, and whole-grain breads.

Remember that, although EVOO is a source of healthy fats, it's also high in calories. Like all fats, at 120 calories per tablespoon, the benefits of EVOO can take a backseat to calorie overload if you overdo it. Buy an oil-misting spray bottle or one with a small pouring spout, or measure out your EVOO by the teaspoon. You might be surprised at how little you actually need.

NEW FINDING

Extra-Virgin Olive Oil May Help Improve Symptoms of Depression

Consuming extra-virgin olive oil (EVOO) may help ease symptoms of severe depression, according to researchers in Iran. Study participants were 73 adults (ages ranging from 28 to 53) randomized to consume 25 milliliters (roughly five teaspoons) of either extra-virgin olive oil (EVOO) or sunflower oil (control group) per day for 52 days. Symptoms of depression were assessed using standardized questionnaires. The study results suggested that consuming EVOO was linked with reduced symptoms of depression in people with severe symptoms, but not with mild or moderate symptoms.

Journal of the Academy of Nutrition and Dietetics, August 2021

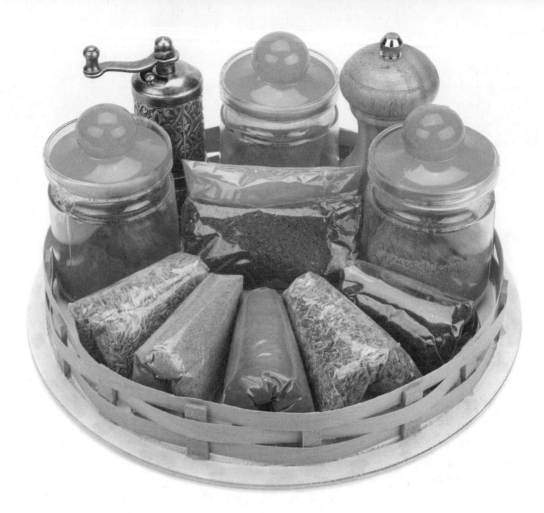

Punching up the flavor of foods with herbs and spices can help you reduce your sodium (salt) intake.

8 Herbs, Spices, and Dark Chocolate

Herbs and spices are compounds that enrich the recipes they're used in; they can enliven the flavor profile of even the most mundane, bland foods.

Herbs are the leaves of a plant, such as basil, parsley, thyme, or oregano, and spices are any other part of the plant, such as the buds, bark, roots, berries, or stigmas (cloves, nutmeg, and peppercorns are examples). Historically, the use of herbs and spices to promote health is well-documented. Over the past centuries, cultures worldwide have recognized a variety of health benefits that can be accessed by exploring the world of herbs and spices.

Researchers have found that phytochemicals in spices and herbs are responsible for some of their powerful antioxidant, antimicrobial, anti-viral, anti-cancer, cholesterol-lowering, kidney- and liver-protecting, and anti-inflammatory properties. In fact, one study showed that adding a blend of spices to meals high in fat and carbohydrates may help lower levels of inflammatory markers, which are substances that indicate inflammation is present.

In the study, all of the participants ate the same high-saturated fat, high-carbohydrate meal, but they consumed varying amounts of a spice blend (including basil, bay leaf, black pepper, cinnamon, coriander, cumin, ginger, oregano, parsley, red pepper, rosemary, thyme, and turmeric) along with the meal. The participants consumed no spice blend (0 grams), 2 grams (about one-third teaspoon) of spice blend, or 6 grams (about one teaspoon) of spice blend. The levels of inflammatory markers were lower in the participants who consumed 6 grams of the spice blend but remained the same in the 2-gram and 0-gram groups.

Health Special Report

PO BOX 8545
BIG SANDY TX 75755-8545

BELSRIR

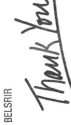

Thank You!

every day and consumers like yourself need an accurate, up-to-date source of reliable information.

That's why we're proud to present you with the updated, Superfoods 2023. In this just published volume, you'll find the latest news and information on practical strategies you should consider.

As announced in the postcard we sent you last month, the price of the new edition remains the same as you paid for last year's edition. We're certain it will be a welcome addition to your home medical library, and we wish you continued good health.

Thanks!

92061300229 HSR008

Health Special Report

PO Box 8545
Big Sandy, TX 75755

#92061300229#   HSR00800016
ANDERSON BARTLETT
1286 HUDSON AVE
SAINT HELENA CA 94574-1920

Packing Slip/Invoice

AMOUNT DUE	INVOICE DATE
$28.90	12/17/22

Qty	Item #	Description
1	SR4523	Superfoods

HSR92061300229008000160002 8900

SFGCONTFFP

Dear Anderson Bartlett,

Smart Seasonings

Herbs and spices provide flavor, fragrance, and color without any of the unwanted "extras" that can accompany other flavor- and texture-enhancing ingredients. Additionally, many herbs and spices contain powerful compounds, with potential benefits including blood sugar regulation, supporting brain function and memory, and soothing gastrointestinal discomfort and nausea. Several herbs and spices are also purported to have anti-inflammatory, antioxidant, and anticancer properties. The easiest way to ensure you're getting maximum benefits is to include a variety of herbs and spices in your meals.

One of the most important health benefits that may be gained by using herbs and spices is helping you lower your sodium intake. The average daily sodium intake for Americans is 3,400 milligrams (mg)—far more than the 2,300 mg (roughly equivalent to one teaspoon of table salt) recommended by the *Dietary Guidelines for Americans*. The American Heart Association goes even further, advising an ideal daily sodium intake of no more than 1,500 mg.

The evidence from hundreds of high-quality studies is clear: There is a direct link between higher sodium intake and high blood pressure, or hypertension. Hypertension, in turn, is a major risk factor for heart disease and stroke. For the estimated 90 percent of Americans who consume excess sodium each day, finding ways to eat less sodium is critical for improving their health.

Sodium- or salt-free herbs and spices contribute flavor, which allows home cooks to reduce or eliminate the amount of salt they use without sacrificing taste.

Get started by stocking a variety of herbs and spices in your spice cabinet, or grow fresh herbs in a window or backyard garden. Sprinkle cardamom, cinnamon, or nutmeg into your breakfast cereal or even your coffee or iced tea.

Snip fresh (or sprinkle dried) green herbs such as basil, oregano, cilantro, parsley, rosemary, tarragon, chives, sage, or thyme over your vegetable omelet, leafy green salad, minestrone soup, yogurt dip, roasted vegetables, or grilled fish. Stir aromatic spices, such as turmeric, paprika, cayenne, or cumin, into soups and chili, whole-grain pasta or pilaf, Asian or Indian dishes, or homemade hummus. Here are commonly available herbs and spices to keep in your pantry:

- Allspice
- Anise
- Basil
- Bay leaf
- Caraway seed
- Cardamom
- Celery seed
- Chervil
- Chives
- Cilantro
- Cinnamon
- Cloves
- Coriander
- Cumin
- Dill weed
- Fennel seed
- Garlic
- Ginger
- Marjoram
- Mint
- Mustard seeds
- Nutmeg
- Oregano
- Parsley
- Pepper
- Poppy seeds
- Rosemary
- Saffron
- Sage
- Tarragon
- Thyme
- Turmeric
- Vanilla

Include a variety of tasty herbs and spices in your diet every day—these are *all* superfoods.

Flavor Boosters

From allspice to vanilla, the world of herbs and spices is rich in diversity, offering an abundant range of sweet, savory, and spicy flavors and aromas. However, some of these seasonings have received more scientific study than others; highlighted below are a few that have exhibited health-promoting properties in clinical trials that are worth celebrating in your diet.

Pepper

Black pepper is probably sitting on your kitchen counter right now, ready to add that gently spicy bite and balance to

Consuming Chili Pepper Linked to Reduced Mortality Risk

Regular intake of chili pepper is associated with a wide range of health benefits, including lower all-cause, cardiovascular, and cancer-related mortality (death), according to results from a comprehensive systematic review that included studies from Iran, China, Italy, and the United States. Researchers who conducted the analysis found that all-cause mortality was 8 to 17 percent lower among those who regularly consumed chili pepper (with consumption of regular consumers ranging from weekly to four or more times per week) than among rare consumers or non-consumers. Other research has suggested that consuming chili peppers has anti-obesity, anti-inflammatory, antioxidant, anticancer, and blood glucose-regulating effects. Additional studies are needed to explore the mechanisms by which chili pepper may beneficially influence mortality rates, as well as the amount of chili pepper that is associated with the most benefit.

American Journal of Preventative Cardiology, March 2022

© Kenishirotie | Dreamstime

Turmeric is the spice that gives many Indian and Asian dishes their rich, golden color.

just about every savory dish on your menu. One of the world's most frequently used spices, black pepper comes from a woody vine that grows in tropical climates. After the small flowers appear, they develop into berries that are called peppercorns, which vary in color depending on their stage of development and processing. Black pepper owes its pungent taste to its main phytonutrient, piperine, which has been linked with antioxidant, anti-inflammatory, and anticancer actions.

Ground red pepper is from a completely different plant—it's made from the dried fruit pod of the *Capsicum* family, which includes several spices, such as chili pepper, tabasco pepper, African chiles, paprika, and cayenne pepper. The common denominator of all of these types of red pepper is their heat, which is produced by its phytonutrient capsaicin, which has anticancer, anti-inflammatory, pain-relieving effects, and it may help reduce mortality risk (see "Consuming Chili Pepper Linked to Reduced Mortality Risk").

Including chili pepper in your diet may even help increase longevity. A recent review of health and dietary records of more than 570,000 people in the U.S., Italy, China, and Iran were used to examine death rates among participants who consumed chili pepper and those who rarely or never did. Compared to those who rarely or never consumed chili pepper, those who did had a 26 percent reduction in cardiovascular deaths, a 23 percent reduction in cancer deaths, and a 25 percent reduction in death from all causes.

If you don't care for spicy foods, use just a pinch or two of pepper to enhance the flavors in your favorite dishes. Try black or red pepper in any savory dish, such as grain-based side dishes, fish and poultry marinades, bean dips, chili, and salt-free seasoning blends.

Turmeric

Turmeric is in the culinary spotlight these days, especially in the wellness world. Native to India, turmeric has long been linked with health in the Eastern world; it's been used in traditional and herbal medicine, especially for arthritis and digestive issues. Turmeric root, which comes from the *Curcuma longa* plant, contains curcumin; research has shown this compound has impressive antioxidant and anti-inflammatory effects.

The anti-inflammatory properties of turmeric have been linked to health benefits for a variety of conditions; research suggests that the spice may be helpful in treating inflammatory bowel disease, rheumatoid arthritis, and even cystic fibrosis. It also has been shown to inhibit the growth of certain cancers and to help protect the heart by reducing oxidative stress and lowering cholesterol levels. Research has even linked curcumin to the management of exercise-induced muscle soreness.

Turmeric's ability to be absorbed by the body is not high, but when ingested with piperine, the active ingredient in black pepper, its availability is significantly improved. A 2021 study reported that supplementation with curcumin and black pepper may help with blood sugar control in people with type 2 diabetes. Study participants diagnosed with type 2 diabetes took a daily supplement consisting of 500 milligrams of curcumin and 5 milligrams of piperine or a placebo for four months. Those who took the supplement with curcumin and piperine had lower blood sugar and triglyceride levels, compared to blood sugar and triglyceride levels in the placebo group, supporting the growing body of evidence for the health benefits of curcumin and piperine.

Perhaps the most exciting news about curcumin is its potential role in the fight against Alzheimer's disease, a condition that is far less prevalent in

India, where turmeric is a key ingredient in many dishes, than it is in Western nations. Research suggests that turmeric may help inhibit the aggregation of beta-amyloid plaques in the brain—a hallmark of Alzheimer's disease. And another study found that turmeric may be helpful in treating depression, but more research is needed before turmeric's possible health benefits are fully understood.

Turmeric is an essential ingredient in traditional Indian dishes, such as dal, masala, and vegetarian dishes that feature other superfoods like cauliflower, chickpeas, lentils, and spinach. Its flavor is versatile enough that you can add it to warm up the flavor and color of your favorite vegetable soup or stew, sprinkle it over roasted vegetables sauté or rice dishes, blend it into smoothies, or add it to tea. Fresh turmeric root is becoming more available in markets; this knobby root can be peeled and sliced into soups, salads, marinades, and vegetable sautés for a burst of color and flavor.

Basil

Basil brings its unique, fragrant appeal to everything it touches. Classic dishes that feature basil include Italian pesto (basil, pine nuts, garlic, olive oil, and Parmesan cheese), Caprese salad (fresh tomatoes and mozzarella topped with basil leaves and drizzled with olive oil and balsamic vinegar), and tomato basil soup. Dive into different cultures' star dishes, like Thai curries and Vietnamese pho (broth-based noodle soups), or toss fresh basil leaves onto any green salad.

There are more than 60 varieties of basil, each with its own unique flavor, aroma, color, and texture; some of the most popular varieties include sweet basil, cinnamon basil, dark opal basil, holy basil, and Christmas basil. Basil is one of the easiest herbs to grow in a pot in the warm months, or keep basil plants inside near a sunny window.

Beyond good taste, basil has been used in some countries as a traditional medicine to help reduce cholesterol levels. While research on basil's health properties is limited, preliminary studies suggest that this herb has lipid-lowering, anti-inflammatory, anti-bacterial, and anticancer properties that are likely related to its numerous phytochemicals, which include eugenol, orientin, and vicenin. Fresh basil also contains vitamins A and K and manganese.

Add fresh basil leaves to sandwiches, scrambles, and flatbreads, chop basil into pasta salads, marinara sauces, and herbal iced tea blends, or top sliced tomatoes or strawberries with basil and drizzle with balsamic vinegar and extra-virgin olive oil for a simple salad. While dried basil is not quite as flavorful as fresh, keep it on hand to flavor bean soup, pasta sauce, marinades, whole-grain stuffing, and roasted vegetables.

Cinnamon

Warm and comforting, cinnamon is considered one of the world's favorite spices. Cinnamon has been used as a flavoring, medicine, embalming agent, and preservative for centuries. Once rare and highly sought after, this fragrant spice, which comes from the inner bark of the cinnamon tree, is widely used in many traditional foods across the globe.

Cinnamon is primarily grown in India, Sri Lanka, Madagascar, Brazil, and the Caribbean. Cinnamon is often considered a sweet spice because it is frequently paired with cakes, muffins, cookies, and fruit pies, and it can boost a dish's flavor enough to allow for less sugar. Cinnamon also adds a fabulous flavor to savory globally inspired dishes, such as Ethiopian stews, North African tagine, and Asian rice and noodle dishes.

Cinnamon has anti-inflammatory, antioxidant, and antimicrobial effects that are related to cinnamon's phytochemicals, which include cinnamyl acetate, cinnamaldehyde, and cinnamyl alcohol, according to clinical research. In addition, cinnamon may help control glucose levels: Cinnamon has been found to slow the rate of stomach emptying, which slows the rise of blood glucose that occurs after eating starches and sugars. And cinnamon may help boost the body's responsiveness to insulin (called insulin sensitivity), which can help manage and control diabetes. Try adding cinnamon to your diet throughout your day: Sprinkle it in your granola, whole-grain porridge, or coffee cup, use it in seasoning blends to sprinkle on fish, add it to savory bean and vegetable stews, and mix it into rice pudding, low-fat yogurt, energy or protein bars, and fruit crisps and cobblers.

Garlic

Garlic has universal appeal for its raw, bold pungency as well as its cooked, caramelized sweetness. One of the most distinctive members of the *Allium* vegetable family, which also includes onions, leeks, scallions, and shallots, this central Asia native has built a reputation as a culinary and medicinal star. Ancient cultures used this pungent bulb to aid heart function and digestion and improve physical strength. Today, garlic is best known as a potent powerhouse that enlivens the flavor and nutrition of any dish.

Every clove of garlic is packed with a variety of sulfur-containing phytochemicals, such as allicin, alliin, and dithiin. In addition, it contains manganese, vitamins B_6 and C, and selenium. These compounds have anti-inflammatory and antioxidant effects, showing promise in lowering cholesterol and blood pressure levels and helping to prevent blood clotting. Garlic also has antibacterial and antiviral effects, which might help fight infections. And, garlic may aid in cancer prevention, specifically against gastric, colorectal, and renal cancers.

While evidence indicates that garlic has health-promoting properties, it has received overly enthusiastic praise from some sources for its ability to treat disease that has not been confirmed in rigorous studies. Don't substitute garlic for traditional heart and cancer treatments recommended by your physician.

Garlic is a mainstay in just about every food culture around the world, from Asia and Europe to the Mediterranean and Central America. A head of garlic contains many separate cloves; remove the papery covering, press or mince the cloves, and stir them into dishes to impart flavor, aroma, and potential health attributes. A clove or two of garlic can flavor sauces, sautés, marinades, dressings, side dishes, vegetables, soups, and pasta dishes. If you find raw garlic too pungent, roast some garlic cloves or an entire head of garlic (cut the top off to expose the cloves) in the oven until the cloves are lightly browned and soft; roasting brings out a sweet, mellow taste. For maximum flavor and nutrition, it's best to start with fresh garlic. However, other convenient forms are available, such as powder and paste, which can be used easily in many dishes.

Ginger

The spiciness of ginger is one of the most unique and well-loved flavors around the world. This knobby root has been celebrated as part of both culinary and healing traditions for centuries, starring in favorite recipes like ginger tea, Indian curries, the pickled accompaniment to sushi, and, of course, gingerbread. The flavorful part of the ginger plant is the underground rhizome, which contains yellow, white, or red-colored flesh with a brown outer skin. Ginger has been used in folk medicine to treat gastrointestinal conditions, and modern science has revealed some evidence-backed benefits in this health arena.

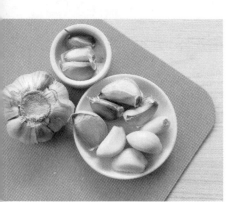

© Juanjalvarezc | Dreamstime

When buying garlic, select heads that are firm, with no soft spots or blemishes. Store garlic in a cool, dark, dry location; refrigeration is not recommended. Garlic can also be stored in the freezer.

Ginger has anti-inflammatory and antioxidant actions possibly related to its phytochemicals called gingerols, which are responsible for ginger's unique flavor. Studies show that ginger may be effective in preventing nausea associated with motion sickness and pregnancy. In addition, ginger has shown promise in relieving pain resulting from arthritis, as well as tumor-fighting activity in animal studies.

Fresh ginger root is available in the produce section of most supermarkets; if you can't find it there, check Asian or Indian food markets. Use ginger by simply peeling and finely grating it into your dishes—or you can use minced, ground, dried, or crystallized ginger. Try adding it to a pot of oatmeal with pears and stirring it into iced tea and sparkling water. Ginger is a good match for veggie side dishes, stir fries, soups, and roasted or mashed winter squash or sweet potatoes. Mix with reduced-sodium soy sauce or tamari, olive oil, and garlic and use as a salad dressing or marinade. Definitely add it to baked goods for warming, sweet-smelling bliss. You can add ground or freshly grated ginger to baked goods, such as muffins, quick breads, and fruit and oatmeal bars.

Dark Chocolate

You don't have to feel guilty about loving chocolate: Thanks to nutrition research, dark chocolate has received a vote of approval for its role in protection against chronic diseases.

Chocolate is made from beans harvested from the *Theobroma cacao* tree. Once the beans are removed from their pods, fermented, dried, and roasted, they are ground into cocoa liquor (a non-alcoholic substance). The cocoa liquor can undergo further processing to produce cocoa butter and cocoa powder, and sugar and vanilla can be added to cocoa liquor to make chocolate. Dark chocolate contains larger amounts of cocoa solids and smaller amounts of sugar than milk chocolate, which results in its rich, deep flavor.

Cocoa beans and dark chocolate are packed with flavanols, the main type of phytochemical that has been linked to protection against heart disease, diabetes, dementia, and stroke. The nutrients in dark chocolate appear to help reduce inflammation, lower blood pressure and cholesterol levels, and protect the heart by improving endothelium function (the endothelium is a layer of cells that lines the heart and blood vessels).

Choose the darkest variety of chocolate possible—at least 70 percent cocoa or cacao—to reap health benefits from chocolate, keeping in mind that the flavanol levels may vary widely among dark chocolate products. (Most scientific studies that have evaluated the effects of dark chocolate consumption have used chocolate with a 70 percent or higher cocoa content.) Milk chocolate has much lower levels of flavanols, and white chocolate has none.

However, even dark chocolate can contribute to extra inches around your waist if it's eaten in excess, counteracting any of its potential health benefits. Every ounce of dark chocolate contains about 170 calories and 12 grams of fat, so savor this healthy indulgence in moderation. Use chopped dark chocolate instead of packaged milk or semi-sweet chips in baking, or melt it to use as a dip for fresh fruit.

You also can use cocoa powder as a low-fat, low-calorie addition to beverages, puddings, granola, and baked goods—one tablespoon contains all of the health potential of dark chocolate, but with just 12 calories and less than 0.5 grams of saturated fat. Cocoa powder has savory as well as sweet applications; use it to add more depth to sauces (think of the Mexican tradition of mole), stews, and seasoning mixes.

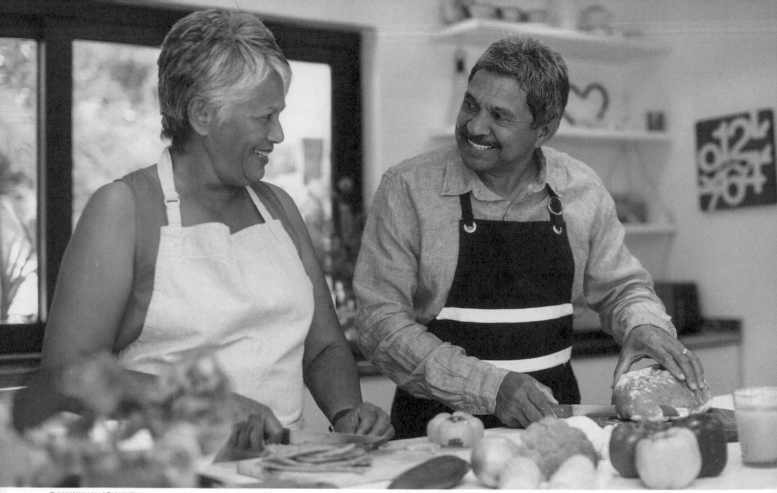

© peopleimages | Dreamstime

Planning ahead is an essential strategy for healthier eating. It's much easier to cook at home when you have plenty of nutritious foods in your fridge, freezer, and pantry.

9 Prepping and Cooking

Congratulations! You've gotten this far and you've now gained considerable knowledge on the health-promoting power of superfoods. It's now time to discuss how to get them into play in your day.

Unfortunately, at the time of writing this report, we are still dealing with the presence of COVID-19, though the overall outlook has been improving. Many people are still utilizing drive-through restaurants and takeout options for meals, which often consist of highly processed foods high in calories, fat, and sodium. As another option, consider the use of home delivery meal service kits. These kits, subscription-based or pay-by-usage, can compile fresh meal choices and fill them with many of the superfoods noted in this report, offering a healthier way to get your superfoods.

Research also shows that cooking at home can have a positive impact on weight loss. In a recent study, participants received either hands-on cooking lessons with a chef, or watched a demonstration of the meal preparation. The group who got hands-on lessons lost significantly more weight (7.3 percent) compared to the demonstration-only group (4.5 percent). Weight loss in the hands-on cooking group met or exceeded six-month averages in similar weight-loss programs without a cooking component. Ultimately, when you do your own cooking, you control exactly what does—and doesn't—go into your meals.

Practical Strategies

As with many things in life, having a plan can be a useful tool for achieving your goals. There are many easily implemented steps and tips that can make healthier meal preparation a reality. Review the following suggestions to see which ones will work best for you. From there, choose your favorite tips to create your own tailored plan.

Make a meal plan each week. A sure-fire strategy for healthful eating is to do some prep work before you set foot in the supermarket. One of the first priorities in mapping out meals for the week is to consider the upcoming week—how busy will you be? When will you be able to set aside time to do food prep? What kinds of meals do you want to eat? Taking all of these points into consideration, create your own personal meal plan for the week. Use this plan to build a grocery list (see "Superfoods Shopping List" on page 78) to ensure that the ingredients are available and ready for you when they are needed. If you prefer using electronic devices, choose a meal-planning and/or grocery-planning app to streamline your weekly meal plans.

Create a shopping list. Use your weekly menu to generate your shopping list, making sure to check for and include basic shelf-stable ingredients, such as dried herbs and spices and canned goods you will need on hand. Then, add fresh items to your list, keeping in mind the seasonal availability of produce. If you're serving the same vegetables and fruits every week, check out your community farmers market for some fresh, seasonal ideas—or even start your own vegetable garden. Don't shy away from frozen or canned produce (choose those with no added ingredients, like sugar and sodium), which are healthy (if not healthier) alternatives to fresh. With a well-stocked pantry and freezer, you can always put a healthy meal together.

Let your kitchen guide you. If you're struggling to come up with ideas for healthy meals, survey your kitchen for inspiration and direction. Check your freezer stash, open the refrigerator, make a visual sweep of the pantry, and let creativity be your guide. Say you have some shrimp in the freezer, broccoli and carrots in the refrigerator, and brown rice and almonds in the pantry. Turn this into a quick stir-fry: Sauté the shrimp, broccoli, and carrots with some herbs and spices, serve over brown rice, and sprinkle with chopped almonds.

Take shortcuts. Keep convenient, healthy items on hand to reduce prep time and get meals on the table quickly. Pre-chopped onions and bell peppers, shredded cabbage and carrots, cubed butternut squash, minced garlic in a jar, frozen vegetable blends, canned, unsalted tomatoes and beans, and bagged, pre-washed salad greens are readily available in markets.

Keep snack packs on hand. Having a stash of healthy superfoods on hand makes it easy to drive past the drive-thru and bypass the office donut box. Store a bag of peanuts or sunflower seeds in your desk drawer, pack sliced cucumbers, radishes, and hummus in a cooler bag, prepare a homemade mix of dried cherries, apricots, and walnuts, or energy bars filled with whole grains and nuts, or take along whole-wheat crackers or pita bread and nut butter.

Put healthy foods within easy reach. Place a large bowl of seasonal fresh fruit on the counter and keep ready-to-eat veggie snacks, like fresh salsa or hummus, snap peas, celery sticks, zucchini wedges, and broccoli and cauliflower florets where you'll see them as soon as you open your fridge. Designate a healthy snack shelf in your pantry or cupboard and stock it with unsalted mixed nuts, a variety of dried fruit, homemade trail mix, and canned fruit or fruit cups (in juice rather than in syrup, which is a form of added sugar).

© Paulmaguire | Dreamstime

It's simple but true: Keeping fruits and other nutritious foods within easy reach means you're more likely to include them in your diet.

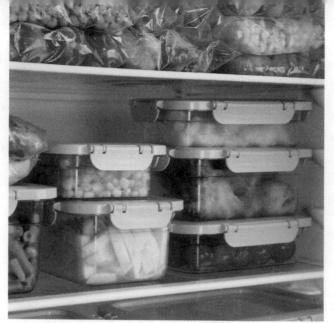

Keeping your freezer stocked with a variety of vegetables means you'll always have access to nutritious choices at mealtime.

Food Prep and Storage

Make the most of your superfoods once you've completed your food shopping by choosing preparation and storage methods that preserve their powerful vitamins, minerals, and phytochemicals.

Fresh is best, frozen is next. Fresh, ripe produce in season usually will be highest in nutrients—but you need to eat fruits and vegetables year-round, even in the middle of winter. According to the U.S. Department of Agriculture (USDA), freezing produce immediately after harvesting retains 95 to 100 percent of most vitamins and minerals, with the exception of vitamin C, which diminishes by up to 30 percent in frozen produce. If fresh fruits and vegetables have traveled a long way to reach your location and/or have been stored for more than a few days, they begin to lose some of their nutrient content, so frozen options may sometimes have a health advantage.

Keep canned on hand. Turn to canned fruits, vegetables, beans, and fish that contain no added sodium or sugar for easy, economical, and convenient meals. Keeping a variety in your pantry or cupboards guarantees you immediate access to important nutrients you need. Research shows that people who include more canned produce in their diets have overall better diets that are higher in important nutrients, such as fiber, vitamin A, calcium, magnesium, and potassium, and lower in saturated fat.

Preserve nutrients. Up to 50 percent of the vitamin C, thiamin, vitamin B_6, and folate content in food can be lost to the water it's cooked in, according to data from the USDA. To retain water-soluble nutrients, use cooking methods like steaming, roasting, grilling, or stir-frying that use little or no water, reduce the amount of water used in steaming, and reuse cooking water in soups or sauces to make use of escaped nutrients.

Make the most of your microwave. Since it cuts cooking time and water use, consider your microwave as a nutrient-friendly kitchen appliance. Microwaving better preserves antioxidant activity in a majority of vegetables compared to other cooking methods, according to research. But be sure to choose glass or ceramic plates and bowls for microwave use; potentially harmful chemicals may leach out of plastic into your food, and some plastics actually begin to break down during microwaving.

Keep it cool. The nutrient content in many fruits and vegetables can be maintained with cooler temperatures and less air contact. Store produce in airtight containers in the fridge to preserve those nutrients.

Don't peel off nutrients. Keeping peels on foods such as sweet potatoes, carrots, cucumbers, apricots, and apples preserves more nutrients, which tend to concentrate near the surface. In place of peeling, opt for a good vegetable scrubber.

Use the whole plant. Next time you get ready to throw away those celery or carrot tops, think again. Many vegetables are entirely edible and rich in nutrients, so use the entire plant to add nutrients to your day and avoid needless food waste. Or toss vegetable scraps into a pot of water and make your own flavorful stock, which can be stored in the freezer and used as a base for soups, stews, and sauces.

Now it's time to start putting the power of superfoods together on your plate. Plan your meals around the healthy proteins, whole grains, vegetables, fruits, unsaturated fats, and herbs and spices you have learned about in the previous chapters. Every meal should contain a balance of each of these food groups. To create meals that meet your optimal nutrient needs, use USDA's MyPlate as a resource. This pictorial guide can quickly steer you to the basics needed for building a healthy meal. Visit the MyPlate website at myplate.gov to learn about the amounts of foods in each category you need to consume each day to protect and preserve your health. You can also download the Start Simple with MyPlate app on your phone for an easy-to-use tool to set daily healthy eating goals, record what you've eaten, and stay motivated by seeing your progress in real time.

Control Portion Sizes

One of the most important strategies for healthy eating and living is simply keeping your portions under control, even if the foods you're eating are healthy. In today's world, big portion sizes are everywhere, from restaurants and fast food drive-thrus to food and beverage packages. In addition, most people significantly underestimate how much food and calories they actually consume—a fact that's been borne out by scientific research. By being more mindful of what and how much you are actually eating, you can scale back your portion sizes and maintain a healthy weight.

Be more mindful of your food intake by eating meals at a dining table rather than eating while working, watching TV, or surfing the internet. Dish up foods on smaller salad plates rather than large dinner plates, and avoid eating straight out of large containers, such as jars of trail mix or boxes of snack foods. Use visual cues to become more aware of standard portion sizes (see page 77 for "A Visual Guide to Portion Sizes").

🔟 Superfoods Recipes

Creamy Edamame and Avocado Dip

Ingredients

2 cloves garlic

¼ cup fresh cilantro, packed

1½ cups shelled edamame (green soybeans)

Juice of ½ of 1 lime

¼ tsp kosher salt

⅛ tsp black pepper

½ of 1 large avocado, pitted

½ cup 2% plain Greek yogurt

2 Tbsp extra-virgin olive oil

Steps

1. Combine the garlic and cilantro in the bowl of a food processor; pulse until very finely chopped.
2. Add the remaining ingredients except the olive oil to the bowl; process until thoroughly combined and smooth.
3. Pour in the olive oil gradually while the motor is running.
4. Transfer to a bowl and garnish with cilantro. Serve as a dip with whole-grain chips, crackers or pretzels, or use as a spread for sandwiches.

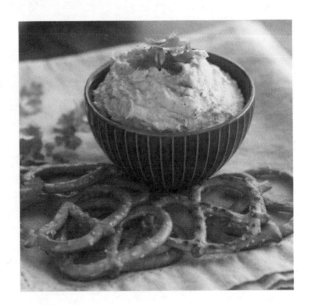

Yield: 5 (¼-cup) servings

Per serving: 124 calories, 10 g fat, 1 g sat fat, 7 g protein, 7 g carbs, 3 g fiber, 1 mg cholesterol, 112 g sodium, 2 g total sugar, 0 g added sugar

Source: Recipe (adapted) and photo reprinted from *The High Protein Vegetarian Cookbook: Hearty Dishes that Even Carnivores Will Love.* ©2015 by Katie Parker and Kristen Smith. Used with permission of The Countryman Press, a division of W.W. Norton & Company, Inc.

Vanilla Brown Sugar Almond Butter

Ingredients

3 cups unsalted roasted almonds

2 tsp vanilla extract

1 Tbsp lightly packed dark brown sugar

¼ tsp fine sea salt

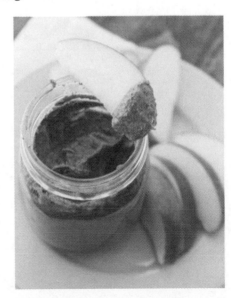

Steps

1. Place almonds in a large food processor or high-powered blender. Process on low for 5 minutes, then boost up to high. Process until smooth; this may take another 10 minutes or more, depending on your food processor's size and power.
2. Add the vanilla, sugar, and salt to the almonds and pulse a few times to combine.
3. Store in an airtight container in the refrigerator for up to 5 days. Serve on whole-grain toast or with fruit, like sliced apples or pears.

Yield: 14 (2-Tbsp) servings

Per serving: 181 calories, 16 g fat, 1 g sat fat, 7 g protein, 7 g carbs, 4 g fiber, 0 mg cholesterol, 35 g sodium, 2 g total sugar, 1 g added sugar

Source: Recipe (adapted) and photo reprinted from *The High Protein Vegetarian Cookbook: Hearty Dishes that Even Carnivores Will Love.* ©2015 by Katie Parker and Kristen Smith. Used with permission of The Countryman Press, a division of W.W. Norton & Company, Inc.

Roasted Garlic Butternut Squash Hummus

Ingredients

1 medium-sized butternut squash (2 pounds), peeled, seeded, and cut into 1-inch cubes

4 cloves garlic

2 Tbsp extra-virgin olive oil, divided

1 Tbsp dried rosemary

1 (15-oz) can chickpeas, drained and rinsed

1 tsp paprika

1 tsp chili powder

¼ tsp ground cayenne pepper

¾ tsp fine sea salt

¾ cup part-skim ricotta cheese

Steps

1. Preheat oven to 400°F.
2. Place butternut squash and garlic on a 9 x 13-inch baking sheet; drizzle with 1 tablespoon olive oil and stir until evenly coated.
3. Wrap the garlic cloves in a small piece of aluminum foil; place the packet of foil on the baking sheet. Sprinkle the dried rosemary over the squash. Bake for 25–30 minutes, until the squash is fork tender; set aside and allow to cool.
4. In a food processor, combine squash, garlic, chickpeas, paprika, chili powder, cayenne, salt, and pepper, and process until smooth. While processor is running, pour in the remaining olive oil.
5. Add the ricotta and process again until smooth.

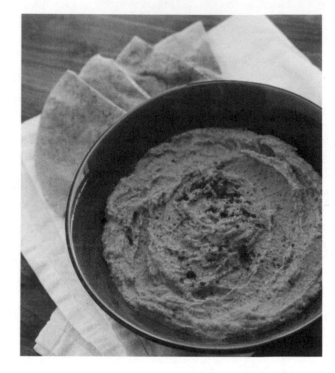

Yield: 8 (⅓-cup) servings

Per serving: 156 calories, 6 g fat, 2 g sat fat, 7 g protein, 20 g carbs, 5 g fiber, 7 mg cholesterol, 259 mg sodium, 3 g total sugar, 0 g added sugar

Source: Recipe (adapted) and photo reprinted from *The High Protein Vegetarian Cookbook: Hearty Dishes that Even Carnivores Will Love.* ©2015 by Katie Parker and Kristen Smith. Used with permission of The Countryman Press, a division of W.W. Norton & Company, Inc.

Fresh Veggie Quinoa Salad with Lemon-Tahini Dressing

Quinoa Salad Ingredients

½ Tbsp extra-virgin olive oil

2 cloves garlic, minced

½ red onion, chopped, divided

1 cup quinoa, uncooked

¼ tsp salt

3 Tbsp fresh thyme, chopped

1 zucchini, diced

1 red pepper, diced

1 tomato, diced

1 (15-oz) can chickpeas, rinsed and drained

⅓ cup raw, unsalted slivered almonds, toasted
      if desired

Lemon-Tahini Dressing Ingredients

¼ cup tahini (sesame seed paste)

¼ cup water

¼ cup lemon juice

1 clove garlic

¼ tsp kosher salt

⅛ tsp freshly ground pepper

½ Tbsp extra-virgin olive oil

Steps

1. Heat the olive oil over medium heat in a large saucepan. Add garlic to the pan and cook until fragrant, stirring frequently, for one minute.

2. Add half of the onions and cook until translucent. Pour in the quinoa and toast for 2–3 minutes, then add 2 cups water, salt, and thyme. Bring to a boil, reduce to low, cover, and simmer for 15 minutes.

3. For the dressing, pulse the tahini, water, lemon, garlic, salt and pepper in a food processor until smooth. Slowly add the olive oil while the processor is running.

4. Add the chopped vegetables (including the remaining raw red onions), chickpeas, and almonds to the cooked quinoa. Pour the dressing over the quinoa mixture; stir until dressing is evenly distributed and serve.

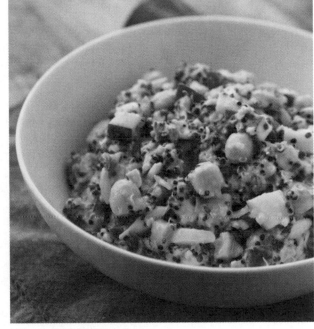

Yield: 5 (about 1¼-cup) servings

Per serving: 279 calories, 13 g fat, 2 g sat fat, 10 g protein, 33 g carbs, 5 g fiber, 0 mg cholesterol, 279 mg sodium, 5 g total sugar, 0 g added sugar

Chunky Potato and Lentil Soup

Ingredients

2 Tbsp unsalted butter

3 cloves garlic, minced

2 shallots, sliced

3 stalks celery, chopped

2 large carrots, peeled and finely chopped

2 russet potatoes, peeled and chopped into
   ½-inch cubes

2 tsp garbanzo bean flour

1 cup water

4 cups no-salt-added vegetable broth

1 (28-oz) can no-salt-added diced tomatoes

2 cup French green lentils, picked over
   and rinsed

1 tsp ground cumin

1 tsp dried oregano

⅛ tsp fine sea salt

¼ tsp ground white pepper

½ tsp red pepper flakes

2 bay leaves

1 Tbsp Dijon mustard

Steps

1. Heat the butter in a large pot over medium-low heat. Stir in the garlic and cook for 30 seconds, and then add the onions and salt and cook for 2–3 minutes, until translucent and soft.

2. Pour in the celery, carrots, and potatoes. Cook for about 10 minutes, until all vegetables are softened.

3. Whisk the garbanzo bean flour into the water until fully dissolved. Add the flour/water mixture, vegetable broth, tomatoes, lentils, spices, and bay leaves into the pot. Reduce to low, cover, and simmer for 45 minutes.

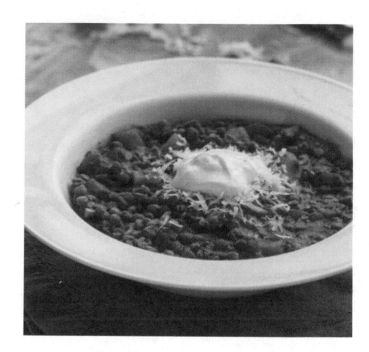

4. Remove bay leaves from the soup, then stir in the dijon mustard.

5. Serve with whole-grain crackers or toast.

Yield: 6 (1½-cup) servings

Per serving: 321 calories, 5 g fat, 2 g sat fat, 20 g protein, 51 g carbs, 11 g fiber, 10 mg cholesterol, 574 mg sodium, 7 g total sugar, 0 g added sugar

Source: Recipe (adapted) and photo reprinted from *The High Protein Vegetarian Cookbook: Hearty Dishes that Even Carnivores Will Love.* ©2015 by Katie Parker and Kristen Smith. Used with permission of The Countryman Press, a division of W.W. Norton & Company, Inc.

Tomato, Barley, and White Bean Soup

Ingredients

3 Tbsp extra-virgin olive oil

3 cloves garlic, minced

½ large yellow onion, chopped

½ cup sundried tomato halves, chopped

1 Tbsp unbleached all-purpose flour

1 Tbsp water

1 (28-oz) can no-salt-added crushed tomatoes

1 (28-oz) can no-salt-added fire-roasted diced tomatoes

2 cups no-salt-added vegetable broth

1 cup 1% milk

2 Tbsp herbs de Provence

1 Tbsp dried rosemary

½ tsp ground white pepper

¼ tsp ground black pepper

¼ tsp crushed red pepper

⅛ tsp fine sea salt (or to taste)

2 tsp granulated sugar

1 (15-oz) can no-salt-added navy beans, rinsed and drained

1 cup pearl barley, uncooked

Steps

1. Heat olive oil over medium heat in a large soup pot or Dutch oven. Add garlic and cook for 30 seconds, stirring frequently to prevent burning. Add onions and cook until translucent (2–3 minutes), stirring occasionally.

2. Add sundried tomatoes and cook until softened for another 2–3 minutes.

3. Whisk together the flour and water. Add the flour mixture, crushed tomatoes, diced tomatoes, broth, milk, spices, sugar, beans, and barley to the soup pot. Taste and adjust seasonings to your liking. Cover and simmer on low for 25–30 minutes, until the barley is tender.

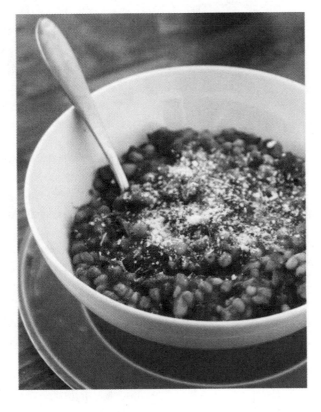

Yield: 6 (1½-cup) servings

Per serving: 344 calories, 9 g fat, 1 g sat fat, 11 g protein, 59 g carbs, 13 g fiber, 2 mg cholesterol, 659 mg sodium, 16 g total sugar, 1 g added sugar

Source: Recipe (adapted) and photo reprinted from *The High Protein Vegetarian Cookbook: Hearty Dishes that Even Carnivores Will Love*. ©2015 by Katie Parker and Kristen Smith. Used with permission of The Countryman Press, a division of W.W. Norton & Company, Inc.

Chipotle, Bean, and Wheat Berry Chili

Ingredients

½ cup wheat berries, uncooked

3 Tbsp extra-virgin olive oil

2 cloves garlic, minced

1 small red onion, diced

3 celery stalks, chopped

1 green pepper, diced

1 red pepper, diced

½ (7.5-oz) can chipotle peppers in adobo sauce

4 cups no-salt-added vegetable stock

1 (28-oz) can no-salt-added diced tomatoes

1 (24-oz) jar or can no-salt-added tomato purée

⅛ tsp kosher salt

¼ tsp black pepper

1 Tbsp chili powder

2 tsp cumin

½ Tbsp dried oregano

1 (15-oz) can no-salt added pinto beans, drained and rinsed

1 (15-oz) can no-salt added dark red kidney beans, drained and rinsed

1 (29-oz) can no-salt added corn, drained and rinsed

Steps

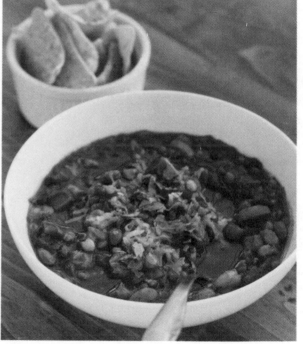

1. In a medium-sized saucepan, bring the wheat berries and 1½ cups water to a boil. Cover, reduce heat to low, and simmer for one hour, or until liquid is absorbed and wheat berries are soft.

2. Heat the oil in a large saucepan over medium heat; add the garlic and cook until fragrant, stirring frequently, for about one minute. Add the onions and cook until translucent, about 3–5 minutes.

3. Drain the can of chipotle peppers; reserve a couple tablespoons of the adobo sauce for later use. Reserve half of the peppers for another use. Cut the remaining peppers in half; use a spoon to scoop out the seeds, and roughly chop the peppers.

4. Add the celery, green peppers, red peppers, and chipotle peppers to the onions; let the veggies cook down for 5–7 minutes, until softened.

5. Add the broth, tomatoes, tomato purée, salt, pepper, spices, beans, and corn to the vegetable mixture; stir until thoroughly combined.

6. Taste the chili and adjust the spices to your liking. If you prefer more spice, add a tablespoon or two of the adobo sauce. Reduce the heat to low, cover, and simmer for at least 30 minutes (or until the wheat berries are cooked).

7. When ready to serve, mix the cooked wheat berries into the chili. Top with cilantro and/or shredded cheese, if desired, and serve with tortilla chips.

Yield: 8 (1¾-cup) servings

Per serving: 334 calories, 7 g fat, 1 g sat fat, 14 g protein, 59 g carbs, 13 g fiber, 0 mg cholesterol, 192 mg sodium, 14 g total sugar, 0 g added sugar

Peanut Butter and Banana Baked Oatmeal

Ingredients

1½ cups old-fashioned oats
1 tsp ground cinnamon
¼ tsp ground nutmeg
½ tsp baking powder
⅛ tsp salt
2 medium overripe bananas

⅓ cup creamy peanut butter
1 cup 1% milk
3 Tbsp maple syrup
½ Tbsp vanilla extract
1 egg

Steps

1. Preheat the oven to 375°F. Coat an 8 x 8-inch baking dish with nonstick spray.
2. Combine the oats, cinnamon, nutmeg, baking powder, and salt in a bowl. Set aside.
3. In another bowl, mash the bananas well, then whisk in the peanut butter, milk, maple syrup, vanilla, and egg.
4. Whisk the dry ingredients into the wet ingredients until well combined. Pour into an 8 x 8-inch baking dish.
5. Bake for 35–40 minutes, until golden on top and set.
6. Let sit for three minutes, then slice into four pieces. Serve warm with additional milk if desired.

Yield: 4 servings

Per serving: 323 calories, 14 g fat, 3 g sat fat, 11 g protein, 42 g carbs, 5 g fiber, 44 mg cholesterol, 217 mg sodium, 22 g total sugar, 9 g added sugar

Source: Recipe (adapted) and photo reprinted from *The High Protein Vegetarian Cookbook: Hearty Dishes that Even Carnivores Will Love.* ©2015 by Katie Parker and Kristen Smith. Used with permission of The Countryman Press, a division of W.W. Norton & Company, Inc.

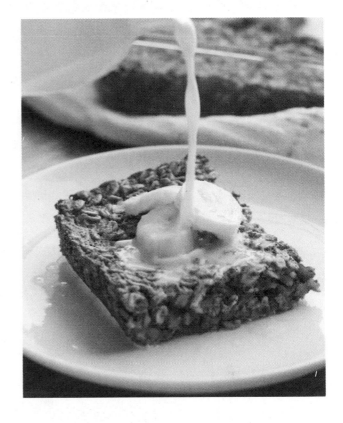

Three-Bean Quinoa Taco Salad

Three-Bean Quinoa Salad Ingredients

1 cup quinoa

2 cups no-salt-added vegetable broth

1 cup black beans, drained and rinsed

1 cup white kidney beans, drained and rinsed

1 cup garbanzo beans, drained and rinsed

2 Roma tomatoes, diced

6 oz (about 4 cups) chopped Romaine lettuce

½ cup fresh cilantro, chopped (can add more for garnish if desired)

1 avocado, cubed

Cilantro-Lime Vinaigrette Ingredients

¼ cup fresh cilantro

¼ of one yellow onion, chopped

1 Roma tomato, seeded and chopped

1 Tbsp white wine vinegar

Juice of 1 lime

2 cloves garlic

1 tsp dried oregano

¼ tsp fine sea salt

¼ tsp ground black pepper

½ tsp ground cumin

¼ tsp paprika

2½ Tbsp extra-virgin olive oil

Steps

1. Combine the quinoa and vegetable broth in a medium-sized pot over medium heat. Bring to a boil; cover and reduce to a simmer for 15–20 minutes, until all liquid is absorbed.

2. While the quinoa cooks, make the dressing. Combine all ingredients except olive oil in a food processor. Process until all ingredients are very finely chopped. Slowly drizzle in the olive oil with the processor running.

3. Combine the cooked quinoa, beans, tomatoes, Romaine, and cilantro in a large bowl. Pour in the dressing and toss thoroughly.

4. Divide into 6 bowls; top with avocado and additional cilantro immediately before serving. Serve with tortilla chips, if desired.

Yield: 6 (2-cup) servings

Per serving: 328 calories, 10 g fat, 1 g sat fat, 15 g protein, 47 g carbs, 9 g fiber, 0 mg cholesterol, 419 mg sodium, 5 g total sugar, 0 g added sugar

Source: Recipe (adapted) and photo reprinted from *The High Protein Vegetarian Cookbook: Hearty Dishes that Even Carnivores Will Love.* ©2015 by Katie Parker and Kristen Smith. Used with permission of The Countryman Press, a division of W.W. Norton & Company, Inc.

Broccoli- and Barley-Stuffed Bell Peppers

Stuffed Peppers Ingredients

1 cup pearl barley, uncooked

3 cups no-salt-added vegetable broth

4 large bell peppers

1 Tbsp extra-virgin olive oil

2 cloves garlic, minced

2 shallots, diced

½ tsp kosher salt

1½ cups broccoli florets, stems removed and roughly chopped

1 cup grape tomatoes, quartered

½ cup fresh basil leaves, chopped

½ cup shredded mozzarella

4 oz fresh mozzarella, sliced

Marinara Sauce Ingredients

2 Tbsp extra-virgin olive oil

1 clove garlic, minced

1 (28.2-oz) can no-salt-added crushed tomatoes

½ tsp kosher salt

¼ tsp crushed red pepper

2 Tbsp chopped fresh basil

½ Tbsp brown sugar

Steps

1. Combine the barley and broth in a saucepan, and bring to a boil over high heat. Reduce heat to low and simmer, covered, for 40–45 minutes.
2. Preheat oven to 350°F.
3. Cut the peppers in half; scoop out the seeds and ribs. (If you keep the top of the stem on, it helps keep the filling from spilling out.)
4. Bring a large pot of water to a boil. Add the peppers, bring the water back up to a boil, and cook for 3 minutes. Remove peppers from the pot; set aside and allow to drain.
5. Heat the olive oil in a large pan over medium heat. Add the garlic and cook until fragrant (about 30 seconds). Add the shallots and salt; cook for 2–3 minutes. Add the broccoli and grape tomatoes, and cook until the broccoli is bright green and the tomatoes are starting to get soft (about 5 minutes).
6. Transfer broccoli mixture to a large bowl. Add the cooked barley, shredded mozzarella, and basil; stir gently to combine.
7. Place the boiled peppers in a 9 x 13-inch baking dish filled with ½ cup of water. Stuff each pepper with filling. To make the most of the filling, push the filling down into the pepper and allow it to heap over the top of the pepper. Top each pepper with a slice of fresh mozzarella; bake for 35 minutes.
8. While peppers are baking, make the sauce. Heat the olive oil over medium heat; add the garlic and cook until fragrant. Add the tomatoes, red pepper flakes, fresh basil, and brown sugar. Bring to a boil, then reduce to a simmer and let cook for 15 minutes.
9. When the peppers are done baking, pour the sauce over the peppers; top with more fresh basil (if desired).

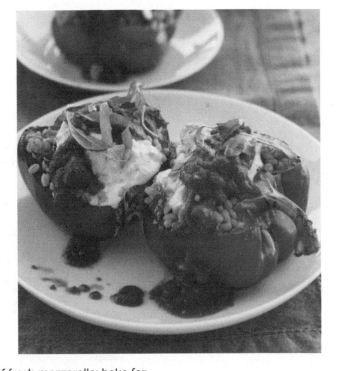

Yield: 8 servings (½ of 1 pepper)

Per serving: 278 calories, 11 g fat, 4 g sat fat, 10 g protein, 36 g carbs, 9 g fiber, 18 mg cholesterol, 458 mg sodium, 10 g total sugar, 0 g added sugar

Buffalo Chickpea Salad Sandwich

Ingredients

1 (15-oz) can garbanzo beans,
    rinsed and drained

¼ cup 2% plain Greek yogurt

1 Tbsp Buffalo-style hot sauce, such as Frank's

2 oz (about ¼ cup) goat cheese, crumbled

1 tsp dried dill

2 cloves garlic

½ tsp Dijon mustard

⅛ tsp fine sea salt

¼ tsp chili powder

½ tsp paprika

⅛ tsp cayenne (or more to taste)

1 Tbsp extra-virgin olive oil

¼ of one red onion, diced

8 slices whole-wheat bread

2 medium tomatoes, sliced

Basil, fresh or dried (optional)

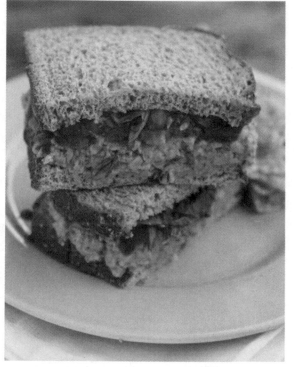

Steps

1. In a large bowl, use a fork to smash the garbanzo beans.

2. In a food processor, combine the yogurt, Buffalo sauce, goat cheese, dill, garlic, mustard, and spices. Process until smooth. Add the oil while the processor is running.

3. Add onion to the beans; pour yogurt sauce over onions and beans, and stir until combined.

4. Divide the chickpea mixture between 4 slices of bread. Top with tomatoes, basil (if desired), and the remaining bread.

5. Cut sandwiches in half and eat as is, or grill in a panini press.

Yield: 4 servings (2 slices of bread and ⅓ cup buffalo chickpea salad per serving)

Per serving: 401 calories, 13 g fat, 5 g sat fat, 21 g protein, 51 g carbs, 11 g fiber, 16 mg cholesterol, 495 mg sodium, 10 g total sugar, 0 g added sugar

Source: Recipe (adapted) and photo reprinted from *The High Protein Vegetarian Cookbook: Hearty Dishes that Even Carnivores Will Love.* ©2015 by Katie Parker and Kristen Smith. Used with permission of The Countryman Press, a division of W.W. Norton & Company, Inc.

Spaghetti and Lentil-Walnut "Meatballs"

Lentil-Walnut Meatballs Ingredients

2 slices whole-wheat bread, toasted

½ cup black lentils, rinsed

1 (15-oz) can navy beans, rinsed and drained

5 oz sliced shiitake mushrooms

½ cup raw, unsalted walnuts, chopped

2 cloves garlic

½ tsp fine sea salt

¼ tsp onion powder

2 Tbsp grated Parmesan cheese

½ cup fresh basil, chopped

½ cup fresh parsley, chopped

1 large egg, lightly beaten

¼ cup whole-wheat flour

16 oz whole-wheat spaghetti, uncooked

Spicy Basil Marinara Ingredients

2 Tbsp extra-virgin olive oil

2 cloves garlic, minced

1 (28-oz) can no-salt-added crushed tomatoes

½ tsp red pepper flakes

½ tsp fine sea salt

¼ cup fresh basil leaves, chopped

Steps

1. Place the bread in a food processor; pulse until finely chopped. Set aside.
2. Combine the lentils and 1 cup water in a small saucepan. Bring to a boil, then cover, reduce heat to low, and simmer for 25 minutes. Check the lentils frequently and add more water if needed. The lentils are ready when they are tender but not mushy.
3. Combine the lentils and next 9 ingredients (beans through parsley) in a food processor. Pulse several times, scraping down the sides as necessary, until all ingredients are very finely chopped but not puréed. You may need to process the mixture in batches, depending on the size of your processor.
4. Preheat oven to 350°F.
5. Stir the bread crumbs into the lentil/bean mixture. Mix in the egg, and then sprinkle in the flour and stir until thoroughly combined.
6. Scoop out 2 tablespoons of the lentil/bean mixture, shape into a ball, and place on a greased baking sheet. Repeat with remaining mixture until you've made 27 meatballs. Coating the meatballs with cooking spray will help them brown on top.
7. Bake meatballs for 35–40 minutes, until set and golden.
8. While meatballs bake, heat the olive oil in a large saucepan over medium heat. Add the garlic and cook until fragrant, about 1 minute; stir in the tomatoes, red pepper flakes, salt, and basil. Heat until mixture just comes to a boil, then cover, reduce heat to low, and simmer for 20 minutes.
9. Cook the pasta according to package directions; drain.
10. Combine pasta and sauce, divide into 9 servings, and top each serving with 3 meatballs.

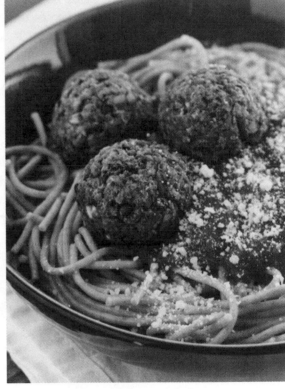

Yield: 9 servings (3 meatballs, ⅓ cup sauce, and ¾ cup spaghetti per serving)

Per serving: 395 calories, 7 g fat, 2 g sat fat, 22 g protein, 64 g carbs, 21 g fiber, 23 mg cholesterol, 508 mg sodium, 9 g total sugar, 0 g added sugar

Source: Recipe (adapted) and photo reprinted from *The High Protein Vegetarian Cookbook: Hearty Dishes that Even Carnivores Will Love.* ©2015 by Katie Parker and Kristen Smith. Used with permission of The Countryman Press, a division of W.W. Norton & Company, Inc.

Sweet-and-Sour Stir Fry with Broiled Tofu

Ingredients

1 Tbsp cornstarch

1 Tbsp water

¾ cup pineapple juice

⅓ cup brown rice vinegar

¼ cup dark brown sugar, packed

3 Tbsp ketchup

1 Tbsp low-sodium soy sauce

1 14-oz block extra-firm tofu, drained and cut into eight 3½ x ½-inch strips

1 Tbsp vegetable oil

2 cloves garlic, minced

1 yellow onion, chopped

½ green onion, chopped

½ red onion, chopped

1 cup brown rice, for serving

Steps

1. Whisk together the cornstarch and water; set aside.
2. Pour pineapple juice, vinegar, sugar, ketchup, and soy sauce into a medium saucepan over medium-high heat; bring to a boil.
3. Reduce heat to medium, whisk in the cornstarch mixture, and cook for another 1–2 minutes, until thickened; set aside.
4. Set the oven to broil.
5. Dip the tofu slices in the sweet-and-sour sauce (the pineapple juice mixture) and place on a greased baking sheet; set the sheet on an oven rack in the upper third of your oven. Broil for 5 minutes, flip, brush with more sweet-and-sour sauce, and broil for another 5 minutes. Flip one more time, brush on more sauce, and broil for 3 more minutes, until the edges have a slight char and the tofu is glossy. Watch the tofu closely as it cooks; there's a fine line between slightly charred and burnt.

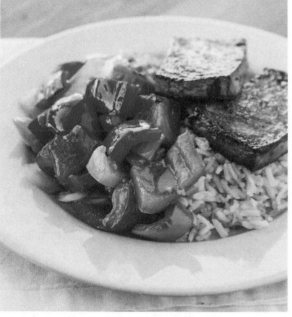

6. While the tofu broils, heat the oil over medium heat in a large skillet. Add the garlic and cook until fragrant, stirring frequently, about one minute. Add onion and cook for 3–5 minutes, stirring occasionally, until softened. Add the peppers and cook for another 5–7 minutes, stirring occasionally, until softened.
7. Cook the brown rice according to package directions.
8. Divide rice into 4 bowls. Top each with one-quarter of the vegetable mixture and 2 slices of tofu.

Yield: 4 servings (¾ cup rice, ¾ cup vegetables, and 2 slices tofu per serving)

Per serving: 414 calories, 9 g fat, 1 g sat fat, 18 g protein, 65 g carbs, 3 g fiber, 0 mg cholesterol, 443 mg sodium, 18 g total sugar, 9 g added sugar

Vegan Roasted Vegetable Lasagna

Filling Ingredients

½ cup roasted unsalted cashews

¼ cup nutritional yeast

2 cloves garlic, chopped

1 tsp dried oregano

1 tsp dried basil

¼ tsp fine sea salt

1 14-oz block extra-firm tofu

Roasted Vegetables Ingredients

1 Tbsp extra-virgin olive oil

1 zucchini, cut into ½-inch pieces

1 red bell pepper, cut into ½-inch pieces

8 oz white mushrooms, sliced

½ of one yellow onion, cut into ½-inch pieces

¼ tsp fine sea salt

¼ tsp ground black pepper

Sauce Ingredients

1 Tbsp extra-virgin olive oil

2 cloves garlic, minced

1 (28-oz) can no-salt-added crushed tomatoes with basil

2 Tbsp tomato paste

½ tsp fine sea salt

1 tsp dried oregano

1 tsp dried basil

¼ tsp crushed red pepper

Assembly Ingredients

8 whole-wheat lasagna noodles

Fresh basil, for garnish (optional)

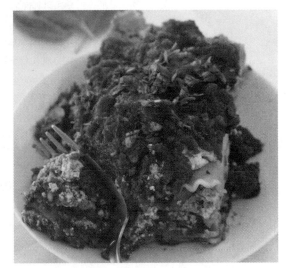

Steps for the filling

1. Place cashews in a small bowl. Pour one cup of boiling water over the cashews; let them sit for 45 minutes.
2. Drain cashews; place them in the bowl of a food processor with the nutritional yeast, garlic, oregano, basil, and sea salt. Process until all ingredients are very finely chopped; transfer the cashew mixture to a bowl.
3. Use your fingers to crumble the tofu; add to the cashew mixture and stir to combine.

Steps for the veggies

1. Preheat oven to 400°F.
2. Combine all vegetables in a bowl. Pour in olive oil and salt, and toss. Spread in one layer on a baking sheet, and roast for 20–25 minutes. Remove from oven; turn oven down to 350°F.

Steps for the sauce

1. Heat the olive oil in a medium saucepan over medium heat.
2. Add the garlic to the pan; cook for 30 seconds, stirring frequently to prevent burning. Add the tomatoes, tomato paste, salt, oregano, basil, and red pepper.
3. Increase heat to medium-high and bring to a boil, then reduce heat to low, cover, and simmer for 15 minutes.
4. Cook lasagna noodles according to package directions.

Steps to assemble

1. Spread ¼ cup of sauce evenly in the bottom of an 8 x 8-inch square baking dish. Top with 2 lasagna noodles. Spread ¼ of the tofu/cashew filling on top of the noodles, ⅓ of the veggies, and ½ cup of the sauce. Repeat this layering twice, then finish with the remaining last 2 noodles, the remaining tofu/cashew filling, and the remaining sauce.
2. Cover with foil; bake for 40 minutes. Remove the foil and bake for another 10 minutes.
3. Let sit for 10 minutes before cutting. Slice into 6 pieces; top with fresh basil, if desired, and serve.

Yield: 6 (about 4" x 2.5" piece) servings

Per serving: 387 calories, 16 g fat, 2 g sat fat, 21 g protein, 44 g carbs, 8 g fiber, 0 mg cholesterol, 468 mg sodium, 11 g total sugar, 0 g added sugar

Source: Recipe (adapted) and photo reprinted from *The High Protein Vegetarian Cookbook: Hearty Dishes that Even Carnivores Will Love.* ©2015 by Katie Parker and Kristen Smith. Used with permission of The Countryman Press, a division of W.W. Norton & Company, Inc.

Wild Rice, Mushroom, and Navy Bean Burgers

Ingredients

½ cup wild rice, uncooked

1½ cups water

3 Tbsp extra-virgin olive oil

3 cloves garlic, minced

½ cup red onion, diced

2 slices whole-wheat bread (roughly 2 cups of breadcrumbs)

4 oz white mushrooms, cut in half

1 (15-oz) can no-salt-added navy beans, drained and rinsed

⅛ tsp cayenne pepper

½ tsp yellow mustard powder

1 Tbsp dried oregano

½ tsp chili powder

½ tsp kosher salt

5 whole-wheat burger buns

Steps

1. Preheat oven to 400°F.
2. In a medium saucepan, bring the water to a boil; add the rice and a sprinkle of salt, reduce heat to low, cover, and cook for 45–50 minutes.
3. Pulse the bread in a food processor until coarse crumbs form.
4. Heat the olive oil in a skillet over medium heat. Add the garlic and cook for 30 seconds. Add the onion and cook until translucent, about 5 minutes. Add the breadcrumbs and cook, stirring frequently, for 2–3 minutes, until lightly browned.
5. Place the mushroom halves in a food processor and pulse until they are finely chopped; set aside.
6. Place the navy beans in the food processor and pulse until mostly smooth.
7. In a large bowl, combine the wild rice, breadcrumb mixture, mushrooms, beans, salt, and spices. Taste and adjust spice level to your liking. Add the egg; mix until well incorporated.
8. Form mixture into 5 patties; place on a baking sheet lined with parchment paper.
9. Bake for 25 minutes, flipping halfway through.
10. Serve on a toasted bun; top with sliced tomatoes and lettuce, if desired.

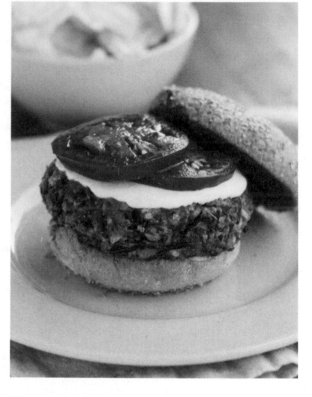

Yield: 5 servings (1 burger each)

Per serving: 372 calories, 12 g fat, 2 g sat fat, 14 g protein, 55 g carbs, 11 g fiber, 37 mg cholesterol, 533 mg sodium, 6 g total sugar, 0 g added sugar

Source: Recipe (adapted) and photo reprinted from *The High Protein Vegetarian Cookbook: Hearty Dishes that Even Carnivores Will Love.* ©2015 by Katie Parker and Kristen Smith. Used with permission of The Countryman Press, a division of W.W. Norton & Company, Inc.

Lemon Millet with Asparagus and Green Peas

Ingredients

1 cup hulled millet, uncooked

2 cups no-salt-added vegetable broth

1½ Tbsp extra-virgin olive oil

¼ cup fresh lemon juice

1½ tsp dried thyme

¼ tsp fine sea salt, divided

20 asparagus spears, tough ends removed, then chopped into 1-inch pieces

1⅓ cup green peas

¼ cup crumbled goat cheese

Steps

1. Preheat the oven to 400°F.

2. Place the millet in a medium saucepan over medium heat and toast for 3–5 minutes, stirring frequently. Add broth, lemon juice, thyme, and half of the salt to the pan, increase heat to medium-high, and bring to a boil. Reduce heat to low, cover, and simmer for 20–25 minutes, until most of the liquid is absorbed. Set aside for 10 minutes; keep covered, so the millet can absorb the remainder of the broth.

3. While millet is simmering, toss the asparagus and green peas together with the olive oil and the remaining salt. Spread evenly on a baking sheet, place in the oven, and bake for 8 minutes; then turn the oven to broil and broil for 2 minutes, until the peas and asparagus are lightly golden.

4. Add asparagus and peas to the cooked millet, sprinkle with goat cheese, and stir gently to combine. Serve while the ingredients are still warm.

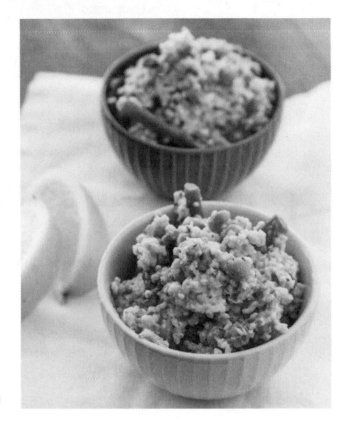

Yield: 6 (¾-cup) servings

Per serving: 217 calories, 7 g fat, 2 g sat fat, 9 g protein, 34 g carbs, 6 g fiber, 4 mg cholesterol, 186 mg sodium, 4 g total sugar, 0 g added sugar

Source: Recipe (adapted) and photo reprinted from *The High Protein Vegetarian Cookbook: Hearty Dishes that Even Carnivores Will Love.* ©2015 by Katie Parker and Kristen Smith. Used with permission of The Countryman Press, a division of W.W. Norton & Company, Inc.

Spanish Quinoa

Ingredients

1 Tbsp extra-virgin olive oil
½ red onion, chopped
1 cup quinoa, dry
1¾ cups low-sodium vegetable broth

1 (14.5-oz) can no-salt-added diced tomatoes
½ cup fresh cilantro, chopped
¼ tsp crushed red pepper

Steps

1. Heat the olive oil in a medium-sized saucepan over medium heat. Add the red onion and cook until softened and translucent (2–3 minutes).
2. Add the quinoa; stir for 2–3 minutes until the quinoa is toasted.
3. Pour in the vegetable broth, tomatoes, cilantro, and red pepper flakes. Bring to a boil; cover and reduce to a simmer for 15–20 minutes, until the liquid is absorbed.

Yield: 4 (1-cup) servings

Per serving: 213 calories, 6 g fat, 1 g sat fat, 7 g protein, 33 g carbs, 4 g fiber, 0 mg cholesterol, 74 g sodium, 4 g total sugar, 0 g added sugar

Source: Recipe (adapted) and photo reprinted from *The High Protein Vegetarian Cookbook: Hearty Dishes that Even Carnivores Will Love.* ©2015 by Katie Parker and Kristen Smith. Used with permission of The Countryman Press, a division of W.W. Norton & Company, Inc.

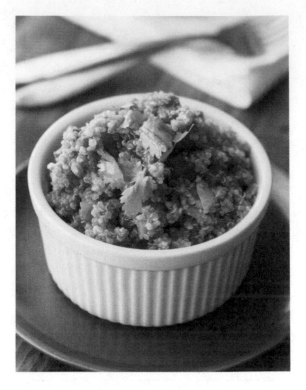

Almond, Cherry, and Quinoa Granola

Ingredients

1 cup quinoa, uncooked

2 cups old-fashioned rolled oats

2 Tbsp chia seeds

¼ cup brown sugar, packed

¼ tsp salt

½ cup slivered raw almonds, unsalted

¼ cup hulled raw pepitas (pumpkin seeds)

½ cup unsweetened flaked coconut

2 Tbsp coconut oil, measured solid

½ cup almond butter (no sugar added)

¼ cup natural applesauce (no sugar added)

3 Tbsp honey

½ tsp almond extract

½ cup dried cherries, unsweetened

Steps

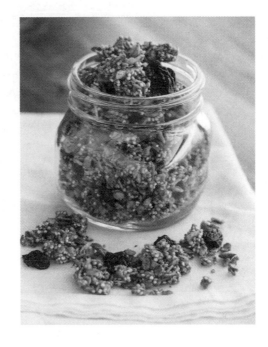

1. Preheat oven to 300°F.
2. Mix together the quinoa, oats, chia seeds, brown sugar, salt, almonds, pepitas, and coconut in a large bowl.
3. In a microwave-safe bowl or in a small saucepan over medium heat, melt the coconut oil and almond butter together. Remove from heat and stir in the applesauce, honey, and almond extract.
4. Pour the wet ingredients into the dry ingredients, and stir until the mixture is evenly coated.
5. Transfer to a parchment-lined baking sheet; bake for 30–40 minutes, stirring frequently, until golden brown.
6. Allow to cool completely; stir in the dried cherries.

Yield: 14 (½-cup) servings

Per serving: 295 calories, 18 g fat, 4 g sat fat, 9 g protein, 29 g carbs, 6 g fiber, 0 mg cholesterol, 81 mg sodium, 11 g total sugar, 6 g added sugar

Source: Recipe (adapted) and photo reprinted from *The High Protein Vegetarian Cookbook: Hearty Dishes that Even Carnivores Will Love.* ©2015 by Katie Parker and Kristen Smith. Used with permission of The Countryman Press, a division of W.W. Norton & Company, Inc.

No-Bake Cherry Nut Energy Bites

Ingredients

½ cup raw slivered almonds

½ cup raw chopped walnuts

¼ cup dried, unsweetened dark cherries

¼ cup dried pitted dates (about 6 dates)

¼ tsp ground cinnamon

1 Tbsp natural almond butter with sea salt

Steps

1. Place all ingredients in a food processor and pulse until very finely chopped. Test the mixture by grabbing some of it with your fingers to see if it sticks together. If it still crumbles a bit, keep processing.

2. Scoop out 2 tablespoons of the mixture, and use your hands to press together into a ball. Repeat with remaining mixture. Recipe will make 8 balls total.

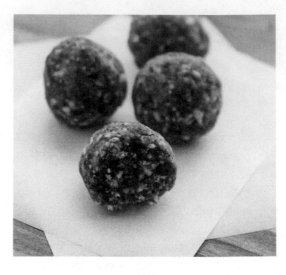

Yield: 4 servings (2 balls per serving)

Per serving: 229 calories, 18 g fat, 1 g sat fat, 7 g protein, 15 g carbs, 4 g fiber, 0 mg cholesterol, 2 mg sodium, 9 g total sugar, 0 g added sugar

Source: Recipe (adapted) and photo reprinted from *The High Protein Vegetarian Cookbook: Hearty Dishes that Even Carnivores Will Love.*

©2015 by Katie Parker and Kristen Smith. Used with permission of The Countryman Press, a division of W.W. Norton & Company, Inc.

A VISUAL GUIDE TO PORTION SIZES

FOOD		PORTION SIZE	VISUAL CUE
Cheese	© Boarding1now | Dreamstime	1¼ ounces	Four Dice
Beef, chicken, fish, pork	© carlosgaw | Getty Images	3 ounces	Deck of Cards
Cooked vegetables	© Bialasiewicz | Dreamstime	½ cup	Baseball
Fresh fruit	© Dshawley | Dreamstime	1 medium	Tennis Ball
Whole grains, pasta, cereal	© Adam Gault | Getty Images	½ cup	Hockey Puck
Raw, leafy vegetables	© Elenathewise | Dreamstime	1 cup	Fist

SUPERFOODS SHOPPING LIST

Clip out this shopping list and take it on your weekly supermarket run. Add your favorite whole foods to each category.

GRAINS
- [ ] Barley
- [ ] Brown rice
- [ ] Bulgur/cracked wheat
- [ ] Oatmeal, old-fashioned or steel-cut
- [ ] Popcorn, light
- [ ] Quinoa
- [ ] Whole-grain bread
- [ ] Whole-grain cereal
- [ ] Whole-grain crackers
- [ ] Whole-grain flour
- [ ] Whole-grain pasta
- [ ] Whole-grain tortillas
- [ ] _____
- [ ] _____
- [ ] _____
- [ ] _____

LEGUMES, NUTS AND SEEDS
- [ ] Almonds
- [ ] Black beans
- [ ] Cannellini beans
- [ ] Chickpeas (garbanzo beans)
- [ ] Kidney beans
- [ ] Lentils
- [ ] Peanut butter
- [ ] Peanuts
- [ ] Pine nuts
- [ ] Pinto beans
- [ ] Pistachios
- [ ] Pumpkin seeds
- [ ] Sesame seeds
- [ ] Soybeans/edamame
- [ ] Sunflower seeds
- [ ] Tofu
- [ ] Walnuts
- [ ] _____
- [ ] _____
- [ ] _____
- [ ] _____

OILS
- [ ] Canola oil
- [ ] Corn oil
- [ ] Extra-virgin olive oil
- [ ] Soybean oil
- [ ] _____
- [ ] _____
- [ ] _____

VEGETABLES
- [ ] Arugula
- [ ] Asparagus
- [ ] Beets
- [ ] Bell peppers, green/ red/orange/yellow
- [ ] Broccoli
- [ ] Brussels sprouts
- [ ] Cabbage, green/red
- [ ] Carrots
- [ ] Corn, sweet yellow
- [ ] Green beans
- [ ] Kale
- [ ] Lettuce
- [ ] Mushrooms
- [ ] Onions, green/red/ white/yellow
- [ ] Peas
- [ ] Potatoes, red/white
- [ ] Radishes
- [ ] Squash, summer/winter
- [ ] Spinach
- [ ] Sweet potatoes
- [ ] Swiss chard
- [ ] Tomatoes
- [ ] _____
- [ ] _____
- [ ] _____
- [ ] _____
- [ ] _____
- [ ] _____
- [ ] _____

FRUITS
- [ ] Apples
- [ ] Apricots
- [ ] Avocados
- [ ] Bananas
- [ ] Blueberries
- [ ] Cantaloupe
- [ ] Cherries
- [ ] Cranberries
- [ ] Dried plums (prunes)
- [ ] Figs
- [ ] Grapes
- [ ] Grapefruit
- [ ] Kiwifruit
- [ ] Mangoes
- [ ] Oranges
- [ ] Peaches
- [ ] Pineapples
- [ ] Plums
- [ ] Raisins
- [ ] Raspberries
- [ ] Strawberries
- [ ] Watermelon
- [ ] _____
- [ ] _____
- [ ] _____
- [ ] _____
- [ ] _____
- [ ] _____
- [ ] _____

DAIRY/DAIRY ALTERNATIVES
- [ ] Cheese, reduced-fat
- [ ] Cottage cheese, low-fat
- [ ] Eggs
- [ ] Milk, low-fat or fat-free
- [ ] Plant-based milk (e.g., soymilk, almond milk)
- [ ] Yogurt, low-fat or fat-free
- [ ] _____
- [ ] _____
- [ ] _____
- [ ] _____

BEEF
- [ ] 90–95% lean ground beef
- [ ] Bottom- or top-round roast or steak
- [ ] Filet mignon
- [ ] Sirloin tip side steak
- [ ] Top sirloin steak
- [ ] _____
- [ ] _____

PORK
- [ ] Tenderloin
- [ ] Boneless loin roast
- [ ] _____
- [ ] _____

FISH AND SHELLFISH
- [ ] Clams
- [ ] Cod
- [ ] Flounder
- [ ] Grouper
- [ ] Halibut
- [ ] Herring
- [ ] Mackerel
- [ ] Mussels
- [ ] Oysters
- [ ] Rainbow trout
- [ ] Salmon
- [ ] Sardines, canned in olive oil or water
- [ ] Scallops
- [ ] Shrimp
- [ ] Tuna (bluefin, yellowfin, skipjack)
- [ ] Tuna, light, canned in water
- [ ] _____
- [ ] _____
- [ ] _____
- [ ] _____

POULTRY
- [ ] Skinless chicken breast
- [ ] Skinless ground chicken or turkey breast
- [ ] Skinless turkey breast
- [ ] _____
- [ ] _____
- [ ] _____
- [ ] _____

alpha-linolenic acid (ALA): An essential fatty acid that, along with EPA and DHA, belongs to a group of fats called omega-3 fatty acids. EPA and DHA are found primarily in fish, while ALA is found in plant seeds and oils, such as flaxseed, canola, soy, walnuts and walnut oils, and in wild plants like purslane. The human body converts a small amount of ALA to EPA and DHA, fatty acids that are linked with a number of health benefits.

amino acids: The building blocks of proteins comprising 20 individual chemical units that are linked together in varying combinations.

antioxidants: Substances that experts believe may protect cells from damage caused by unstable molecules known as free radicals, which are produced by the body as a normal byproduct of metabolism. Antioxidants include flavonoids, beta-carotene, lycopene, selenium, and vitamins A, C, and E.

carbohydrates: Compounds of carbon, hydrogen, and oxygen that form sugars, starches, and celluloses, mostly in plants, which provide energy for the body.

cholesterol: A waxy, fat-like substance found in foods of animal origin and synthesized by the body. Cholesterol is used for many of the body's processes, including hormone production. In large amounts in the blood, cholesterol can clog arteries.

DASH diet: The Dietary Approaches to Stop Hypertension (DASH) eating plan is high in fruits, vegetables, and grains, and low in meat, saturated fat, sweets, and salt. Many studies have shown that you can bring down high blood pressure with this eating plan.

docosahexaenoic acid (DHA): A type of omega-3 fatty acid found in fish that is essential for heart and brain health.

eicosapentaenoic acid (EPA): A type of omega-3 fatty acid found in fish that is essential for heart and brain health.

fats: Compounds containing fatty acids, which may be monounsaturated, polyunsaturated, or saturated.

free radical: A highly reactive atom or compound produced through normal metabolism or from smoking and other toxins. Free radicals damage cell membranes, DNA, and other molecules in the body. They are neutralized by antioxidants.

glucose: A sugar used by the body as a source of energy. For example, food is broken down in the digestive system into glucose.

high-density lipoprotein (HDL) cholesterol: A protein particle that carries LDL ("bad") cholesterol from your tissues to the liver for excretion. HDL is "good" cholesterol and reduces cholesterol buildup in the arteries. High levels of HDL are desirable, because they are linked with a reduced risk of cardiovascular disease that can lead to heart attack or stroke.

lipid: A word used to encompass many different kinds of fat-soluble molecules, including cholesterol, triglycerides, and free fatty acids.

low-density lipoprotein (LDL) cholesterol: A protein particle that carries cholesterol throughout the body. If it builds up in the coronary arteries, it can lead to heart disease. LDL is "bad" cholesterol.

Mediterranean-style diet: A dietary pattern similar to that traditionally found in areas around the Mediterranean Sea in countries such as Greece, southern Italy, and Spain. It emphasizes olive oil as the primary source of dietary fat, an abundance of plant foods, including fruits, vegetables, whole grains, beans, nuts, and seeds, and moderate amounts of fish, poultry, dairy foods, and wine. A Mediterranean-style diet is low in red meat and saturated fats and contains no added sugars or processed foods.

monounsaturated fat: A type of healthy fat in which only one carbon atom is not bound to hydrogen (this is also called a "double bond"); monounsaturated fats, found in olive, walnut, canola, and other vegetable oils, are generally liquid at room temperature.

omega-3 fatty acids: Unsaturated fats found in fish, walnuts, flaxseeds, and some other plant foods that are associated with disease prevention. Diets rich in omega-3s have been linked with a reduced risk of cardiovascular disease and depression, as well as improved brain function.

omega-6 fatty acids: A type of unsaturated fat found in many nuts, seeds, and vegetable oils, and in some poultry, seafood, and vegetables. One omega-6 fatty acid, linoleic acid, is essential because your body requires it but cannot make it, so it must be obtained from your diet.

phytonutrients: Compounds in plants that provide flavor, aroma, and color, and protect the plant from microbes and environmental damage. When consumed by humans, phytochemicals are believed to promote health and prevent disease. Many phytonutrients are antioxidants.

polyunsaturated fat: A type of healthy fat in which more than one carbon atom is not bound to hydrogen; polyunsaturated fats found in soybean, corn, sunflower, and other vegetable oils are generally liquid at room temperature.

protein: An essential component of all living cells. Dietary protein supplies the body with essential amino acids needed for the formation, growth, and repair of cells and tissues in muscles, bones, blood, and skin, as well as the production of enzymes and hormones.

saturated fat: A type of fat that can increase unhealthy cholesterol levels and raise the risk of heart disease. Saturated fatty acids are found primarily in animal foods, especially meats and full-fat dairy products.

triglycerides: A form of fat found in food, fat tissue, and the bloodstream; calories you consume that are not used immediately by the body's tissues are converted to triglycerides and transported to fat cells to be stored. Elevated triglycerides in the bloodstream are a risk factor for heart disease.

unsaturated fat: A type of fatty acid that lowers cholesterol levels and reduces the risk for coronary artery disease especially when it is consumed in place of saturated and trans fats. Monounsaturated and polyunsaturated fatty acids fall into this category.

whole grains: Grains that contain all the essential parts and naturally occurring nutrients of the entire grain seed—the bran, germ, and endosperm.

Academy of Nutrition and Dietetics
800-877-1600
www.eatright.org

Alzheimer's Association
800-272-3900
www.alz.org

AARP
888-687-2277
www.aarp.org

American Cancer Society
800-227-2345
www.cancer.org

American Diabetes Association
800-342-2383
www.diabetes.org

American Institute for Cancer Research (AICR)
800-843-8114
www.aicr.org

American Heart Association (AHA)
www.heart.org
800-242-8721

Centers for Disease Control and Prevention (CDC)
800-232-4636
www.cdc.gov

Environmental Working Group
202-667-6982
www.ewg.org

Food and Drug Administration (FDA)
888-463-6332
www.fda.gov

National Osteoporosis Foundation
800-231-4222
www.nof.org

National Agricultural Library
301-504-5755
www.nal.usda.gov

National Cancer Institute (NCI)
800-422-6237
www.cancer.gov

National Institutes of Health
301-496-4000
www.nih.gov

National Resources Defense Council (NRDC)
212-727-2700
www.nrdc.org

Office of Dietary Supplements
301-435-2920
www.ods.od.nih.gov

Produce for Better Health Foundation
302-235-2329
www.pbhfoundation.org

USDA Center for Nutrition Policy and Promotion
202-720-2791
www.fns.usda.gov/cnpp

USDA Choose My Plate
888-779-7264
www.choosemyplate.gov

The Whole Grains Council/Oldways
617-421-5500
www.wholegrainscouncil.org
www.oldwayspt.org